MANAGEMENT
of the
CARDIAC PATIENT
with
RENAL FAILURE

MANAGEMENT
of the
CARDIAC PATIENT
with
RENAL FAILURE

DAVID T. LOWENTHAL, M. D., F.A.C.P., F.A.C.C.
Professor of Medicine and Pharmacology
Director, Division of Clinical Pharmacology
Likoff Cardiovascular Institute
Hahnemann Medical College and Hospital
Philadelphia, Pennsylvania

RONALD S. PENNOCK, M. D., F.A.C.C.
Associate Professor of Medicine
Co-Director, Department of Critical Care Medicine
Likoff Cardiovascular Institute
Hahnemann Medical College and Hospital
Philadelphia, Pennsylvania

WILLIAM LIKOFF, M. D., F.A.C.C.
Professor of Medicine
President & Chief Executive Officer
Hahnemann Medical College and Hospital
Philadelphia, Pennsylvania

GADDO ONESTI, M. D.
Professor of Medicine and Pharmacology
Division of Nephrology & Hypertension
Department of Medicine
Hahnemann Medical College and Hospital
Philadelphia, Pennsylvania

 F.A.DAVIS COMPANY·Philadelphia

Library of Congress Cataloging in Publication Data
Main entry under title:

Management of the cardiac patient with renal failure.

   Includes index.
   1. Heart—Diseases.   2. Kidneys—Diseases.
I. Lowenthal, David T.   [DNLM: 1. Heart
diseases—Complications.   2. Kidney disease—Complications.   WG 200 M266]
RC682.M29   616.1'2   80-39953

To the patients with the problems herein described
who have provided us with answers

FOREWORD

The kidney has many functions, and dysfunction can have profound effects on cardiovascular activity. Circulatory disturbances in patients with renal failure are common and often life-threatening. It is of prime importance that the clinician be aware of the physiologic interrelation between the kidney and the heart.

In recent years, a better understanding of the pathophysiology of renal failure coupled with new techniques of management has greatly prolonged the survival of patients with advanced renal disease who are managed either conservatively or with chronic hemodialysis. Maintenance hemodialysis for end-stage renal disease has itself evolved dramatically during the past decade.

Most patients with chronic renal failure inevitably experience minor and major cardiovascular complications. It is therefore vital for the physician to recognize these problems in patients with chronic renal disease.

The authors of *Management of the Cardiac Patient with Renal Failure* have addressed themselves to this important medical problem, bringing the associated factors into a sharper focus. The quality of care for these patients will improve if attention is directed to understanding and managing cardiorenal problems in clinical medicine.

Bernard L. Segal, M.D.

PREFACE

Transplantation, peritoneal and hemodialysis have provided modalities for treating end-stage renal disease that significantly prolong life, but subsequently have brought patients to the coronary care unit or sub-acute facility with advanced cardiovascular disease. Answers to the questions raised by this complex clinical presentation are not readily available to the physician. Can one dialyze a patient with acute myocardial infarction? Can bypass surgery be performed? What pharmacologic nuances arise in these patients?

To answer these problems we wrote this book, describing the pathology, physiology and pharmacology of the cardiovascular system in the patient with chronic renal failure. Following these chapters we address more specific clinical problems encountered in the management of cardiac disease in association with end-stage renal failure.

This book was developed from our own practical teaching experience, and we are confident that it will be useful to those facing this growing patient population.

David T. Lowenthal, M.D.
Ronald Pennock, M.D.
William Likoff, M.D.
Gaddo Onesti, M.D.

CONTRIBUTORS

Melton B. Affrime, Pharm. D.

Assistant Professor of Medicine
and Pharmacology
Hahnemann Medical College and Hospital
Philadelphia, Pennsylvania

Gary J. Anderson, M.D.

Professor of Medicine and Physiology
Director, Heart Station
Hahnemann Medical College and Hospital
Philadelphia, Pennsylvania

Arnold R. Eiser, M.D.

Assistant Attending Physician,
Mt. Sinai Service; City Hospital Center at Elmer
Clinical Instructor
Mt. Sinai School of Medicine
New York, New York

Inder P. Goel, M.D.

Associate Professor of Surgery
Department of Cardiothoracic Surgery
Hahnemann Medical College and Hospital
Philadelphia, Pennsylvania

Kwan Eun Kim, M.D.

Professor of Medicine
Head, Renal Laboratory
Hahnemann Medical College and Hospital
Philadelphia, Pennsylvania

Morris N. Kotler, M.D., F.R.C.P.
Professor of Medicine
Director, Echocardiographic Laboratories
Hahnemann Medical College and Hospital
Philadelphia, Pennsylvania

William Likoff, M.D., F.A.C.C.
Professor of Medicine
President and Chief Executive Officer
Hahnemann Medical College and Hospital
Philadelphia, Pennsylvania

David T. Lowenthal, M.D., F.A.C.P., F.A.C.C.
Professor of Medicine and Pharmacology
Director, Division of Clinical Pharmacology
Likoff Cardiovascular Institute
Hahnemann Medical College and Hospital
Philadelphia, Pennsylvania

Lionel U. Mailloux, M.D.
Associate Professor of Clinical Medicine
Cornell University Medical College
Co-Chief, Division of Nephrology and Hypertension
North Shore Hospital
Manhasset, New York

Hugh A. McAllister, M.D., Col. MC, USA AFIP
Armed Forces Institute of Pathology
Washington, District of Columbia

Robert T. Mossey, M.D.
Assistant Professor of Medicine
Cornell University Medical College
Associate Attending Physician
North Shore University Hospital
Manhasset, New York

Eldred D. Mundth, M.D.
Professor of Medicine
Chairman, Department of Cardiothoracic Surgery
Hahnemann Medical College and Hospital
Philadelphia, Pennsylvania

Gaddo Onesti, M.D.
Professor of Medicine and Pharmacology
Division of Nephrology and Hypertension
Department of Medicine
Hahnemann Medical College and Hospital
Philadelphia, Pennsylvania

Wayne R. Parry

Instructor in Medicine
Former Chief Technician, Non-Invasive Laboratory
Hahnemann Medical College and Hospital
Philadelphia, Pennsylvania

Ronald S. Pennock, M.D., F.A.C.C.

Associate Professor of Medicine
Co-Director, Department of Critical Care Medicine
Likoff Cardiovascular Institute
Hahnemann Medical College and Hospital
Philadelphia, Pennsylvania

Andrew R. Schwartz, M.D.

Professor of Medicine
Director, Division of Infectious Diseases
Hahnemann Medical College and Hospital
Philadelphia, Pennsylvania

Stuart Snyder, M.D.

Assistant Professor of Medicine
Hahnemann Medical College and Hospital
Philadelphia, Pennsylvania

Charles E. Swartz, M.D.

Professor and Vice-Chairman
Department of Medicine
Director, Division of Nephrology and Hypertension
Hahnemann Medical College and Hospital
Philadelphia, Pennsylvania

Clifford Wlodaver, M.D.

Fellow in Infectious Diseases
University of Pennsylvania School of Medicine
Philadelphia, Pennsylvania

CONTENTS

1

PATHOLOGY OF THE CARDIOVASCULAR SYSTEM

HUGH A. MCALLISTER, JR., M.D., Col. MC, USA

CARDIOVASCULAR LESIONS INDUCED BY PRIMARY RENAL FAILURE

Myocardial Involvement Secondary to Metabolic Abnormalities

Atherosclerosis is a frequent complication in patients on chronic hemodialysis, usually resulting in either coronary heart disease or cerebrovascular disease, and, indeed, is the major cause of death among these patients.[1] The disorders potentially contributing to earlier and more frequent cardiovascular disease in hemodialysis patients are numerous; probably the most important contributing factor is hypertension (see Chapter 9). The patient with severe hypertension of long duration most likely has preexisting cardiac or cerebral disease or both and is already at risk before the onset of either uremia or hemodialysis. Atherosclerosis is probably accelerated by the well known risk factors of hypertension and also by the metabolic alterations which occur in the uremic patient.

One metabolic alteration that frequently occurs in chronic renal failure is hyperlipidemia (see Chapter 6). *Type IV lipoproteinemia* is the most common form, consisting of a raised triglyceride concentration in whole plasma and in a very low density lipoprotein fraction of plasma.[2] In patients with type IV lipoproteinemia, cholesterol in the whole plasma is normal; however, in those with chronic uremia, cholesterol in the high density lipoprotein fraction is reduced secondary to a deficiency of hepatic lipase.[3-5] Epidemiologic studies have shown that plasma high density lipoprotein concentration is negatively correlated with the risk of acquiring ischemic heart disease.[6] Therefore, high density lipoprotein seems to protect against ischemic heart disease, and the low levels in uremia could be related to accelerated atherosclerosis and the high incidence of heart disease. Many patients with chronic renal disease and type IV hyperlipoproteinemia have impaired fibrinolysis which may be an additional factor in the development of atherosclerosis.

The effectiveness of hemodialysis in controlling the hemostatic abnormalities of uremia is well known. The bleeding time is decreased, ADP-induced platelet aggregation is improved, platelet adhesiveness is increased, and platelet factor 3 activity release is improved following hemodialysis.

During dialysis, however, there is *contact activation of platelets*, and *platelet thrombi* form on dialysis membranes resulting in microemboli. When returned to the patient, these microaggregates may be responsible for the cerebral, renal, or myocardial impairment occasionally observed after coronary bypass surgery, a procedure which also makes use of extracorporeal machines. The adherence of platelet aggregates to damaged endothelium results in release of a mitogenic factor that stimulates proliferation of the intimal smooth muscle cell with subsequent uptake of low density lipoprotein, thus enhancing atherogenesis. Therefore, it is conceivable that by controlling the bleeding tendency or uremic patients by chronic hemodialysis, we have perhaps contributed to accelerated atherosclerosis. Fortunately, recent studies have indicated that platelet aggregation and the subsequent formation of microemboli during extracorporeal circulation can be reversed by using such drugs as aspirin.

Regardless of the precise mechanism of action, the presence of *lipid abnormalities* in patients with uremia on chronic maintenance dialysis most likely contributes to premature and more frequent development of atherosclerosis and mortality from cardiovascular disease.

In addition to the abnormal lipid metabolism in patients with uremia, there is an *abnormal carbohydrate metabolism*.[8,9] Abnormal carbohydrate metabolism has been documented as an early manifestation of the uremic syndrome. This abnormality in carbohydrate metabolism appears to be related to a decreased tissue sensitivity to insulin at the cellular level leading to carbohydrate intolerance. Additionally, there is a delayed and increased release of immunoreactive insulin in uremic patients. Institution of hemodialysis improves this disorder to some extent with reduction of blood glucose and increase in glucose clearance, but fasting and peak immunoreactive levels do not revert to normal. Indeed, immunoreactive insulin levels have been demonstrated to increase in the dialyzed patient, possibly accounting for the improved glucose tolerance.[10] Nevertheless, abnormal carbohydrate metabolism persists to a mild degree in the dialyzed uremic patient and may contribute to the vascular pathology.

Another contributing factor in the development of vascular disease in the uremic patient is *secondary hyperparathyroidism*. *Metastatic calcification* involving the coronary arteries has been well documented in uremic patients and may lead to myocardial fibrosis with congestive heart failure. In addition to calcification of the coronary arteries, there may be myocardial calcification which is particularly ominous when it involves the conduction system. Calcified nodules situated high in the bundle of His may cause complete heart block. In uremic patients, calcification and fibrosis of the sinoatrial and atrioventricular nodes are not uncommon. In the myocardium, metastatic calcification first appears as a fine basophilic granulation in small groups of otherwise morphologically normal myofibers. Later myofiber degeneration becomes apparent, and eventually confluent areas of calcification completely replace large areas of myocardium and are commonly surrounded by dense fibrosis.

Uremia may be a factor influencing the development of multiple minute foci of myocardial necrosis which subsequently calcify. The laws of mass action and of ionic equilibrium of saturated solutions of poorly soluble salts explain, in the case of tricalcium phosphate, the ease with which precipitation may be induced by increases of calcium or phosphate. Massive calcification of the myocardium may be revealed in roentgenograms during the life of a patient.

The *arterial calcification* of hyperparathyroidism characteristically involves the internal elastic membrane and the adjacent media. Although the large elastic arteries (aorta and pulmonary artery) are commonly involved in metastatic calcification, medium sized muscular arteries, as well as arterioles, capillaries, and venules may be involved as well. Metastatic calcification of coronary arteries and arterioles with luminal narrowing is a common finding, and the intimal proliferation associated with this calcification may occasionally be sufficient to cause ischemic myocardial damage. The myocardial and vascular pathology of advanced secondary hyperparathyroidism clearly plays a prominent role in the increased death rate in patients with chronic renal failure.

In addition to myocardial and vascular metastatic calcification, there is suggestive evidence that hyperparathyroidism may contribute to risk factors associated with accelerated atherosclerosis. Hyperparathyroidism seems to have a minor role in abnormal carbohydrate metabolism and a minimal effect on hyperlipidemia.[11] The major pathophysiologic impact of hyperparathyroidism, however, is myocardial and vascular calcification.

In summary, type IV lipoproteinemia with decreased plasma levels of high density lipoprotein, the effects of extracorporeal circulation on platelet aggregation, myocardial and vascular calcification, hypertension, anemia, as well as nutritional, metabolic, and biochemical disturbances may all combine in various degrees to adversely affect the myocardium in the uremic patient on maintenance hemodialysis.

Endocardial Involvement

In addition to myocardial disturbances, uremic patients often have involvement of the endocardium. Valvular calcification due to hyperparathyroidism may follow or accentuate preexisting valvular disease. When valvular calcification occurs in the uremic patient with secondary hyperparathyroidism, the aortic valve is most commonly involved.

Infective endocarditis is more common in the patient with uremia than in the general population (see Chapter 10). Despite apparent adequate maintenance hemodialysis, the uremic patient remains a compromised host, and, indeed, infection is the second most common cause of death in these patients and accounts for approximately 20 percent of all deaths in this population. Impairment of most immunologic defense mechanisms has been documented in uremia, including both impaired delayed hypersensitivity and impaired ability to produce humoral antibody, as well as delayed chemotaxis.[12] Arteriovenous shunts and fistulas are prime sites for entrance of bacteria into the circulation, resulting in septicemia and septic pulmonary embolization, as well as bacterial endocarditis. Although there is an increase in the incidence of involvement of the right sided heart valves in hemodialysis patients, the cardiac valves most commonly involved in bacterial endocarditis are the mitral and aortic valves. Septicemia with or without infective endocarditis most commonly occurs in patients with arteriovenous fistulas or shunts which may or may not appear infected. Although staphylococcus is the most common organism causing bacterial endocarditis in these patients, other less common organisms such as *Serratia marcescens* and opportunistic fungi occur with increased frequency in these immunologically compromised individuals. In addition to infective endocarditis, the patient on chronic hemodialysis who develops disseminated intravascular coagulation may concomittantly develop nonbacterial thrombotic endocarditis which also most commonly is present on the mitral and aortic valves.

Pericardial Involvement

Pericarditis is a frequent occurrence in the uremic patient (see Chapter 5). The incidence in nondialyzed patients is high, with perhaps 40 to 50 percent having pericarditis at some time during their terminal course.

The incidence of pericarditis in most patients on stable chronic hemodialysis is approximately 10 to 20 percent.[13] Uremic pericarditis is usually fibrinous, however, the widespread use of intermittent hemodialysis appears to have increased the incidence of pericardial tamponade and fibrinohemorrhagic pericarditis, perhaps influenced by heparinization or by prolongation of life.

Pathologically, fine mesh-like deposits of fibrin which occur first at the base of the heart in the region of the great vessels cause roughening and thickening of the normally smooth, translucent serous membranes. Serous effusion of variable degree accompanies the fibrinous inflammation. Acute fibrinous pericarditis, if minimal, may resolve completely; if more extensive, the exudate becomes organized and is replaced by fibrous tissue. If the exudate is abundant, the visceral and parietal layers of the pericardium may become bound together by adhesions, or the pericardial cavity may become virtually obliterated by fibrous adhesions. If these fibrous adhesions are extensive, chronic constrictive pericarditis may develop and has been reported to occur as early as 6 weeks and as late as 11 months following acute hemorrhagic pericarditis.[14] When tamponade occurs, it is usually of sudden onset and is frequently precipitated by dialysis. Various reasons for this association of tamponade with dialysis have been proposed, ranging from volume depletion to bleeding associated with heparinization.[13]

The etiology of uremic pericarditis is unknown. Although several theories have been proposed, no one has produced evidence that solidly favors one over another. Yet another consideration in the uremic patient who develops pericarditis is infection. The high incidence of septicemia has been alluded to in these immunologically compromised patients. Virus infections may result in fibrinous pericarditis, whereas bacteria and fungi commonly cause a purulent pericarditis which may occasionally be accompanied by myocardial abscesses. Purulent pericarditis may result in cardiac tamponade or may evolve into chronic constrictive pericarditis. The rare occurrence of tuberculous pericarditis in these patients with impaired delayed hypersensitivity must also be considered in the differential diagnosis.

DISEASES CAUSING SIMULTANEOUS ALTERATIONS IN THE HEART AND KIDNEYS

Collagen Vascular Diseases

Certain generalized diseases are capable of causing lesions in the heart and kidneys independently. Many of the collagen vascular diseases cause pathologic alterations in the heart, as well as the kidney. Those most commonly affecting both of these organ systems include systemic lupus erythematosus, scleroderma, rheumatoid arthritis, panarteritis nodosa, Wegener's granulomatosis, and thrombotic thrombocytopenic purpura.

SYSTEMIC LUPUS ERYTHEMATOSUS

Some type of cardiac abnormality is observed in more than 50 percent of patients with clinical systemic lupus erythematosus (SLE) and in at least that percentage of autopsied cases of SLE.[15] Atypical verrucous endocarditis of Libman and Sacks is recognized as a specific valvular abnormality occurring in SLE and has been encountered in from 25 to 60 percent of autopsied patients.[16] The lesions are small, usually ranging from 1 to 4 mm in diameter, but rarely achieving the size of 8 to 10 mm. They are sterile, dry, granular pink vegetations that may be single or multiple and conglomerate. They have no special tendency to occur along the lines of closure of valves, may be scattered on the endocardium of the valves or on the chordae tendineae, and may also be found on the mural endocardium of the atria or ventricles. Any valve may be involved, but the mitral and tricuspid valves are most often affected. Clinical manifestations of atypical verrucous endocarditis are considerably less frequent than the morphologic lesions observed at autopsy and have been described in 6 to 20 percent of patients with SLE.[17] This discrepancy between the clinical and autopsy incidence of this lesion supports the view that atypical verrucous endocarditis rarely causes significant valvular dysfunction. Histologically, the verrucae consist of a finely granular eosinophilic material which is fibrinoid and may contain hematoxylin bodies. In a general sense, these hematoxylin bodies are the tissue equivalent of the LE cell of the blood and bone marrow. The verrucous endocardial lesions result from degenerative and inflammatory processes of the endocardium and deeper layers of the valves. An intense valvulitis is present which is characterized by fibrinoid necrosis of the valve substance that is often contiguous with the vegetation. Exudative and proliferative cellular reactions are present in the deeper layers of the valve. Healing of these lesions may produce foci of granulation tissue which develop into focal fibrous thickenings in the valves or the mural endocardium. Rarely, bacterial endocarditis has been superimposed on the Libman-Sacks lesion.

Nonspecific interstitial myocarditis has been observed in SLE.[17] The lesions are focal collections of inflammatory cells including polymorphonuclear leukocytes, lymphocytes, plasma cells, and macrophages with interstitial edema and often damage to adjacent myofibers. Occasionally, fibrinoid necrosis is found in interstitial locations, especially adjacent to small blood vessels, and is usually associated with an exudative reaction. Vascular lesions in the myocardium are frequent, with small arteries, arterioles, and venules being principally affected. These vascular lesions consist of fibrinoid changes in the blood vessel walls, varying amounts of inflammatory exudate, and granular or hyaline thrombi in the vessel lumens. Clinically heart failure has been ascribed to the myocardial lesions.

Less well recognized is the occasional report of myocardial infarction in young patients with systemic lupus erythematosus and coronary arteritis.[18,19] In addition to myocardial infarction secondary to arteritis of the extramural coronary arteries in patients with SLE, premature severe atherosclerosis resulting in myocardial infarction has been reported in some of these young women, raising the question as to whether SLE predisposed the patient to early atherosclerosis, possibly as a complication of the arteritis.[20] Another potential factor for accelerated atherosclerosis in these patients is prolonged corticosteroid therapy with its associated alterations in carbohydrate metabolism.

Pericarditis is regarded as the most frequent lesion associated with SLE on the basis of combined clinical and autopsy observations.[15] Most commonly the pericarditis of SLE is fibrinous with or without adhesions. It may or may not be asymptomatic and progression to constrictive pericarditis is rare. Histologically, fibrinoid necrosis with a mixed inflammatory infiltrate and granulation tissue with occasional hematoxylin bodies are present in varying combinations.

Pericarditis with or without effusion has been reported in patients with drug induced SLE. Hydralazine and procainamide have been the drugs most commonly associated with this syndrome. It is rare, however, for patients with drug induced SLE to present with pericarditis as the major initial manifestation, and cardiac tamponade is exceptional.[21]

SCLERODERMA

In scleroderma, myocardial scarring that cannot be attributed to any other cause is the most frequent finding. This myocardial scarring has no particular relationship to blood vessels and cannot be correlated with the presence of vascular intimal lesions which exist in the form of mucoid or fibrinoid degeneration or both and which are even less common in the heart than fibrosis. In contrast to the myocardial lesions of dermatomyositis, there is only minimal infiltration of lymphocytes and plasma cells. Areas of morphologically normal myocardium are interspersed among the foci of fibrosis. Whether or not the myocardial fibrosis is primary or secondary to degeneration of the myofibers has not been established. Although congestive heart failure may result from the myocardial lesions, it is more frequently associated with cor pulmonale secondary to scleroderma or pulmonary disease or to systemic hypertension resulting in left ventricular heart failure.[22]

Nonspecific fibrinous pericarditis, occasionally with a serous effusion, is commonly found at autopsy; however, clinically it is rarely symptomatic. In the patient with scleroderma and renal failure, however, the previously discussed complications of uremic pericarditis must be considered.

Valvular lesions in scleroderma are distinctly rare, but when present the most common lesion is nonbacterial thrombotic endocarditis. The cardiac valves most commonly involved are the mitral and aortic.

RHEUMATOID ARTHRITIS

Approximately 50 percent of patients dying with rheumatoid arthritis will have morphologic evidence of heart disease at autopsy. There is a marked disparity between the incidence clinically and pathologically in that only 10 to 20 percent of these patients with rheumatoid arthritis have fibrous, obliterative pericarditis at autopsy. Rarely, calcific or cholesterol pericardial disease may be present. Usually there are no functional consequences resulting from the obliterative pericarditis; however, a small number of these patients will progress to constrictive pericarditis. The fibrous pericarditis present in these patients is usually nonspecific; however, in approximately 20 percent diagnostic rheumatoid granulomas are present.[23] Rheumatoid granulomas are present in the myocardium in 32 percent of these patients and are most frequently located in the left ventricular myocardium.[23] When they involve the conduction system, varying degrees of heart block may be encountered clinically. In addition to diagnostic rheumatoid granulomas in the myocardium, approximately 10 percent of these patients will have a nonspecific interstitial myocarditis at autopsy. Rheumatoid nodules may also occur, although less frequently, in the cardiac valves. The two valves most commonly affected are the mitral and aortic. Approximately 10 percent of these patients will have rheumatoid granuloma present in epicardial coronary arteries, and in 10 percent the aorta will be involved as well.[23] Coronary artery involvement may lead to myocardial infarction in the absence of atherosclerosis. When the aorta contains rheumatoid nodules they are most commonly located in the proximal 3 cm of the ascending aorta and rarely, if ever, progress to clinically significant sclerosing aortitis.

PANARTERITIS NODOSA

Panarteritis nodosa is a form of necrotizing arteritis that chiefly affects medium sized muscular arteries—the coronary arteries being no exception. The active lesion of panarteritis nodosa consists of segmental necrosis and inflammation of all layers of the arterial wall. The inflammatory cell population is mixed, but in the active lesion polymorphonuclear leukocytes are the most common. Fibrinoid necrosis is usually present in the intima and inner one third of the media, and a superimposed thrombus is frequently encountered. These lesions are usually present in varying stages of evolution and devolution, and the arterial lumen may be occluded by fresh thrombus or by formation of granulation tissue, fibrosis, and recanalization in varying combinations. The myocardial lesions in panarteritis nodosa are usually secondary to involvement of the epicardial coronary arteries, resulting in myocardial infarction. Occasionally, however, there is a nonspecific myocarditis consisting mainly of polymorphonuclear leukocytes with focal myofiber necrosis. Because of the variety of the stages of development of the lesions in the epicardial arteries, the myocardial infarcts will also be of various sizes and in different stages of evolution, ranging from healed infarcts with fibrous scarring to acute myocardial infarction. Other morphologic findings include cardiac hypertrophy and fibrinous pericarditis. In most instances, the cardiac hypertrophy is related to hypertension, whereas the pericarditis may be related to uremia and not to primary cardiac disease. Clinically, the most frequent manifestation of cardiac involvement in panarteritis nodosa is congestive heart failure.[24]

WEGENER'S GRANULOMATOSIS

Wegener's granulomatosis often is confused with panarteritis nodosa, since both of these diseases are characterized by disseminated vasculitis, renal disease, and cardiac disease. As previously discussed, in classic panarteritis nodosa medium sized muscular arteries are involved; in contrast, Wegener's granulomatosis involves predominantly small arteries, arterioles, and venules. In addition, pulmonary arteries are not usually involved in classic panarteritis nodosa, whereas pulmonary disease is common in Wegener's granulomatosis. Necrotizing granulomata and upper airway disease so characteristic of Wegener's granulomatosis are not features of panarteritis nodosa. Cardiac pathology is present in approximately 30 percent of patients with Wegener's granulomatosis at autopsy.[25]

Wegener's granulomatosis can affect the heart in any number of forms, including pericarditis, which is usually fibrinous, pancarditis, or coronary arteritis with acute myocardial infarction. Although fibrinous pericarditis is the most common lesion encountered, myocarditis and coronary arteritis are the most devastating. The clinical manifestations of cardiac involvement include chest pain, intractable arrhythmias, and congestive heart failure.

THROMBOTIC THROMBOCYTOPENIC PURPURA

Thrombotic thrombocytopenic purpura is regarded by many as a collagen vascular disease. This condition is characterized by endothelial damage to arterioles and formation of hyaline deposits which may obstruct these vessels. These vascular lesions are usually widespread throughout the body. Cardiac involvement is secondary to vascular lesions of coronary arterioles, the obstruction of which may lead to focal areas of necrosis of myocardial fibers. Although the most common cardiac involvement in thrombotic thrombocytopenic purpura is focal myocardial necrosis, nonbacterial thrombotic endocarditis is not uncommon. The cardiac valves most commonly involved with nonbacterial thrombotic endocarditis are the mitral and aortic. Embolization from these lesions through the systemic circulation is extremely common.

Metabolic Diseases

In addition to the collagen vascular diseases, some metabolic diseases cause simultaneous structural alterations in both the heart and kidneys. Those metabolic diseases that most commonly affect both of these organ systems include amyloidosis, Fabry's disease, hyperoxaluria, and gout.

AMYLOIDOSIS

Amyloid involvement of the heart occurs in five categories: primary amyloidosis, secondary amyloidosis, familial primary amyloidosis, senile cardiac amyloidosis, and amyloidosis associated with multiple myeloma. Clinical and pathologic investigations reveal a remarkable overlap among the different types of amyloidosis with regard to organ distribution. Whereas the heart is most commonly involved in the primary forms of amyloidosis and the kidney is involved most commonly in secondary amyloidosis and in some of the heredofamilial disorders, particularly familial Mediterranean fever, concomitant involvement of both organs must be considered in any form of amyloidosis.

In cardiac amyloidosis the myocardium is involved more frequently than the pericardium or epicardium. Both the atria and ventricles may be diffusely or focally affected. Most commonly, the interstitium of the myocardium is diffusely infiltrated and the compressed myocardial fibers undergo atrophy or occasionally focal necrosis. Extensive deposition destroys the myofibers entirely, leaving empty amyloid rings or solid sheets of amyloid. The sarcoplasm of atrophic myofibers is vacuolated and contains deposits of lipid or lipochrome pigment. Usually the greater the amount of amyloid in the myocardium, the greater degree of heart failure. Any area of the conduction system may be affected in amyloidosis. The sinus node may be heavily involved, and, therefore, its efficiency as a pacemaker may be impaired. Characteristically amyloid is also deposited in the media of intramyocardial coronary arterioles. Less frequently, there may be amyloid deposits in the extramural coronary arteries, as well as intramural capillaries and veins. On rare occasions amyloid deposits can considerably narrow the epicardial coronary arteries resulting in myocardial infarction.[26] Although the mural endocardium is infiltrated by amyloid in most cases, amyloid deposits in the heart valves are only present in 50 percent of affected patients. Valvular involvement is usually minimal, but occasionally discrete nodules measuring from 1 to 4 mm in diameter are present on the valves, either in the cusp or the annulus. Rarely, valvular involvement is diffuse, resulting in thick, rigid cusps, and stenotic or insufficient orifices. All four cardiac valves are affected with almost equal frequency. Involvement of the pericardium and epicardium may be either nodular or diffuse. Occasionally pericardial amyloidosis may be accompanied by a serous pericardial effusion.

FABRY'S DISEASE

Fabry's disease (angiokeratoma corporis diffusum universale) is an inherited metabolic disease characterized by intracellular accumulation of the neutral glycolipid, ceramide trihexoside. The cause of the disease is a deficiency in the lysosomal enzyme, ceramide trihexosidase.[27] A variety of clinical signs and symptoms develop, usually during childhood, and initially consist of dark purple keratotic lesions in the skin of the trunk, bouts of fever, proteinuria, abdominal pain, disturbances of sweating, and parasthesias in the limbs.

In most male patients, hypertension, edema, cardiac dysfunction, renal failure, and uremia develop during the third and fourth decades of life. Because the disease is transmitted by a sex-linked gene that is variably and incompletely recessive, hemizygotic male patients exhibit the full spectrum of the disease, whereas most heterozygotic female patients develop only corneal dystrophy and some degree of renal involvement. Although reasonable longevity may be expected for most female subjects, full penetrance and premature death may be seen occasionally. Cardiac involvement in Fabry's disease is a constant pathologic feature in affected males and occasionally may be present to a severe degree in affected females.[28]

In addition to the effects of hypertension and uremia on the heart secondary to renal involvement in Fabry's disease, there are extensive glycolipid deposits in the cardiac muscle fibers, vascular smooth muscle, endothelium, and connective tissue cells of the cardiac valves, especially the mitral valve.[28] These glycolipid deposits are present in practically all atrial and ventricular muscle cells, including those of the conduction system.[27] They are especially prominent in the myofibers of the inner-most layers of the ventricular myocardium. Smooth muscle cells of the endocardium and coronary blood vessels, as well as the endothelial cells and perivascular cells, contain small scattered deposits of glycolipid. The glycolipid may be present in histiocytes and other connective tissue cells of the myocardium and the cardiac valves.[28] Deposition of the glycosphingolipid in extramural coronary arteries has occasionally caused luminal compromise of marked degree, resulting in myocardial infarction. More typically, however, there is an electrocardiographic pattern of myocardial infarction secondary to deposition of the glycosphingolipid in myocardial cells with no gross evidence of infarction at autopsy.[27] Other common electrocardiographic abnormalities are atrial fibrillation and varying degrees of heart block ranging to complete heart block. The deposition of glycosphingolipid in the mesenchymal cells of the aorta is frequently accompanied by marked fragmentation of elastic lamellae with the formation of pools of acid mucopolysaccharide. Because of these degenerative lesions in the aorta media, one could expect dissecting aneurysm to complicate the clinical course of the patient with Fabry's disease, especially in view of the frequent occurrence of systemic hypertension. Thus far, this event has not been reported, however.

HYPEROXALURIA

Primary hyperoxaluria is a rare disorder characterized clinically by calcium oxalate nephrolithiasis and nephrocalcinosis, which frequently leads to progressive renal failure and death in uremia. Calcium oxalate deposits frequently occur in extrarenal tissue, including the heart. The pathologic condition is termed oxalosis. The basic defect is an impairment of metabolism of glyoxylic acid, resulting in an overproduction of oxalic acid and consequent precipitation of the insoluble calcium oxalate salt.[29] There is increased urinary excretion of oxalic and glyoxylic acids. In the majority of families the data are consistent with an autosomal recessive pattern of inheritance.[29] Although 65 percent of patients develop symptoms before five years of age, and 90 percent die with a history of symptoms of less than 10 years duration, some patients with primary hyperoxaluria do not follow the classic pattern of onset and progression of the disease.[30] Patients with adult onset primary oxalosis have been described, as have patients with a milder form of the disease.

In this latter group, life expectancy is highly variable. Thus, there is a heterogeneity in both the clinical and biologic features of primary hyperoxaluria. In addition to the adverse cardiac effects of uremia and hypertension in these patients, calcium oxalate crystals are deposited in the myocardium and conduction system leading to myocardial insufficiency, congestive heart failure, and complete heart block. Complete heart block secondary to oxalate deposits in the conduction system occurs most commonly in the classic juvenile onset type of primary oxalosis, but has been described, although rarely, in patients with adult onset primary oxalosis and in oxalosis secondary to renal failure of long duration.[30]

Moderate degrees of hyperoxaluria have been noted in a number of diseases in which calcium oxalate renal stones are occasionally found. These diseases include hepatic cirrhosis, Klinefelter's syndrome, renal tubular acidosis, and sarcoidosis.[29] In none of these disorders has significant oxalate deposition been described in the myocardium. Experimental pyridoxine deficiency and experimental thiamine deficiency cause hyperoxaluria in animals, suggesting that deficiencies of these two vitamins may contribute to oxalosis in humans.[29] Ethylene glycol ingestion results in central nervous system depression, severe metabolic acidosis, acute renal tubular necrosis, and deposition of calcium oxalate crystals in the kidneys and extrarenal tissues. However, death most commonly occurs in the first 48 hours during the phase of severe acidosis, and calcium oxalate crystals are rarely found at autopsy.

GOUT

Gout most commonly affects the heart through its effects on the kidneys resulting in hypertension and/or uremia. Rarely, however, tophi develop in the heart. When they occur, they are usually in the left ventricular endocardium or on the mitral valve.[31] Cardiac tophi are usually asymptomatic and are incidental findings at autopsy. Rarely there has been extension of a tophus into the conduction system resulting in complete heart block.[32] It is conceivable that large tophi on the mitral valve could result in varying degrees of mitral insufficiency.

Hyperuricemia and gout may be associated with an increased incidence of arteriosclerotic cardiovascular disease.[33] In the Framingham study, patients with gout had twice the risk of coronary heart disease as those without it. In hyperuricemic patients without gouty arthritis, the risk of coronary heart disease was not increased. Recent in vitro studies suggest that urate crystals have a role in atherogenesis. Incubation of platelets with monosodium urate crystals results in rapid release of serotonin, adenosine triphosphate (ATP), and adenosine diphosphate

(ADP). ADP is a potent stimulator of platelet aggregation and effects a further release reaction and aggregation. In vivo platelet aggregation may be an important initiating event in atherosclerosis. As compared with a control population, patients with gout and no family history of atherosclerosis have an increased turnover and a decreased half life of platelets.

Idiopathic Arterial Calcification of Infancy

Finally, idiopathic arterial calcification of infancy (juvenile intimal sclerosis) is a rare disease of undetermined etiology, characterized by deposition of calcium salts in the internal elastic membrane and contiguous media associated with intimal hyperplasia, resulting in luminal compromise. These arterial changes are widespread throughout the arteries of the body, with the exception of those of the brain. The arteries most commonly and most severely involved are the coronary arteries, renal arteries, and splenic artery. The aorta and pulmonary artery are affected less frequently. The age of patients dying with this disorder has ranged from 3 days to 28 months, with 85 percent of patients dying within the first six months of life.[34] Myocardial infarction is the most frequent cause of death, and congestive heart failure is the most common presentation, followed by sudden unexpected death. A definite tendency for the disease to occur in siblings has been noted, but additional patterns of inheritance are not yet apparent.[34] There is no apparent sex predilection, and there is no consistent evidence of a metabolic disturbance with calcium or phosphorus.

SUMMARY

Recent epidemiologic data contend that unless ischemic heart disease[35] and/or hypertension[36] exists before the development of renal failure, that accelerated atherosclerosis does not occur in renal failure. This chapter surveys the consequences of the pathologic changes within the cardiovascular system in patients with primary or secondary renal failure regardless of initiating abnormalities. The pathophysiology of hypertension in patients with renal impairment is discussed in Chapter 2.

REFERENCES

1.   Lowrie, E.C., Lazarus, J.M., Mocelin, A.J., et al.: Survival of patients undergoing chronic hemodialysis and renal transplantation, N. Engl. J. Med. 288:863, 1973.
2.   Frederickson, D.S., Levy, R.I., and Lees, R.S.: Fat transport in lipopro-

teins—an integrated approach to mechanisms and disorders. N. Engl. J. Med. 276:34, 1967.

3. Bagdade, J.D., and Albers, J.J.: Plasma high-density lipoprotein concentration in chronic-hemodialysis and renal-transplant patients. N. Engl. J. Med. 296:1436, 1977.

4. Brunzell, J.D., Albers, J.J., Haas, L.B., et al.: Prevalence of serum lipid abnormalities in chronic hemodialysis. Metabolism 26:903, 1977.

5. Rapoport, J., Aviram, M., et al.: Defective high-density lipoprotein composition in patients on chronic hemodialysis. N. Engl. J. Med. 299:1326, 1978.

6. H.D.L. and C.H.D. Lancet 2:131, 1976.

7. Wardle, E.N., Menon, I.S., and Anderson, J.: A study of patients with atherosclerosis and renal disease with respect to lipoprotein types, fibrinolysis, and carbohydrate tolerance. Quart. J. Med. 41:15, 1972.

8. Hampers, C.K., Soeldner, J.S., Doak, P.B., et al.: Effect of chronic renal failure and hemodialysis on carbohydrate metabolism. J. Clin. Invest. 45:1719, 1966.

9. Alfrey, A.C., Sussman, K.E., and Holmes, J.H.: Changes in glucose and insulin metabolism induced by dialysis in patients with chronic uremia. Metabolism 16:733, 1967.

10. Hampers, C.L., Schupak, E., Lowrie, E.G., et al.: Long-Term Hemodialysis, ed. 2. Grune and Stratton, New York, 1973, p. 173.

11. Lazarus, J.M., Lowrie, E.G., Hampers, C.L., et al.: Cardiovascular disease in uremic patients on hemodialysis. Kidney Int. [Suppl.] (2):167 (Jan.), 1975.

12. Baum, J., Cestero, R.V., and Freeman, R.B.: Chemotaxis of the polymorphonuclear leukocyte and delayed hypersensitivity in uremia. Kidney Int. [Suppl.] (2):147 (Jan.), 1975.

13. Marini, P.V., and Hull, A.R.: Uremic pericarditis: A review of incidence and management. Kidney Int. [Suppl.] (2):163 (Jan.), 1975.

14. Comty, C.M., Cohen, S.L., and Shapiro, F.L.: Pericarditis in chronic uremia and its sequels. Ann. Intern Med. 75:173, 1971.

15. Baggenstoss, A.H., and Titus, J.L.: Rheumatic and collagen disorders of the heart, in Gould, S.E. (ed.): Pathology of the Heart and Blood Vessels, ed. 3. Charles C Thomas, Springfield, Ill., 1968, p. 701.

16. Larson, D.L.: Systemic Lupus Erythematosus. Little, Brown, Boston, 1961, p. 26.

17. Brigden, W., Bywaters, E.G.L., Lessof, M.H., et al.: The heart in systemic lupus erythematosus. Br. Heart J. 22:1, 1960.

18. Cheitlin, M.D., McAllister, H.A., and deCastro, C.M.: Myocardial infarction without atherosclerosis. JAMA 231:951, 1975.

19. Bonfiglio, T.A., Botti, R.E., and Hagstrom, J.W.C.: Coronary arteritis, occlusion and myocardial infarction due to lupus erythematosus. Am. Heart J. 83:153, 1972.

20. Tsakraklides, V.G., Blieden, L.C., and Edwards, J.E.: Coronary atherosclerosis and myocardial infarction associated with lupus erythematosus. Am. Heart J. 87:637, 1974.

21. Ghose, M.K.: Pericardial tamponade: A presenting manifestation of procainamide-induced lupus erythematosus. Am. J. Med. 58:581, 1975.

22. Baggenstoss, op. cit., p 705.

23. Robinowitz, M., Virmani, R., and McAllister, H.A.: Rheumatoid heart disease: a clinical and morphologic analysis of 34 autopsy patients. J. Lab. Invest. 42:49, 1980.

24. op. cit., p 707.
25. Fauci, A.S., and Wolff, S.M.: Wegener's granulomatosis and related diseases. Disease-a-Month 23 (7):1, 1977.
26. Brigden, W.: Cardiac amyloidosis. Prog. Cardiovasc. Dis. 7:142, 1964.
27. Brady, R.O., Gal, A.E., and Bradley, R.M., et al.: Enzymatic defect in Fabry's disease. Ceramidetrihexosidase deficiency. N. Engl. J. Med. 276:1163, 1967.
28. Ferrans, V.J., Hibbs, R.G., and Burda, C.D.: The heart in Fabry's disease—a histochemical and electron microscopic study. Am. J. Cardiol. 24:95, 1969.
29. Williams, H.E., and Smith, L.H., Jr.: Primary hyperoxaluria, in Stanbury, J.B., Wyngaarden, J.B., Fredrickson, D.S. (eds.): The Metabolic Basis of Inherited Disease, ed. 3. McGraw-Hill, New York, 1972, pp. 196–219.
30. West, R.R., Salyer, W.R., and Hutchins, G.M.: Adult-onset primary oxalosis with complete heart block. Johns Hopkins Med. J. 133:195, 1973.
31. Batsakis, J.G.: Degenerative lesions of the heart, in Gould, S.E. (ed.): Pathology of the Heart and Blood Vessels, ed. 3. Charles C Thomas, Springfield, Ill., 1968, p. 483.
32. Hench, P.S., and Darnall, C.M.: Clinic on acute oldfashioned gout: with special reference to its inciting factors. Med. Clin. N. Am. 16:1371, 1933.
33. Boss, G.R., and Seegmiller, J.E.: Hyperuricemia and gout—classification, complications and management. N. Engl. J. Med. 300:1459, 1979.
34. Moran, J.J.: Idiopathic arterial calcification of infancy: a clinicopathologic study, in Sommers, S.C. (ed.): Cardiovascular Pathology Decennial 1966–1975. Appleton-Century-Crofts, New York, 1975, pp. 47–71.
35. Rostand, S.G., Gretes, J.C., Kirk, K.A., et al.: Ischemic heart disease in patients with uremia undergoing maintenance hemodialysis. Kidney International 16:600, 1979.
36. Vincenti, F., Amend, W.J., Abele, J., et al.: The role of hypertension in hemodialysis—associated atherosclerosis. Am. J. Med. 68:363, 1980.

2

HYPERTENSION: HEMODYNAMIC ALTERATIONS AND PATHOPHYSIOLOGY

KWAN EUN KIM, M.D., GADDO ONESTI, M.D., AND CHARLES SWARTZ, M.D.

Hypertension is both a cause and a complication of chronic renal disease. A knowledge of the hemodynamic changes in hypertension secondary to renal parenchymal disease is essential for an understanding of the underlying pathophysiologic mechanisms and management.

The hemodynamic factors regulating blood pressure may be expressed in the equation BP = CO × TPR, where BP is the mean arterial blood pressure, CO the cardiac output, and TPR the total peripheral resistance. High blood pressure may result from a high cardiac output or a high total peripheral resistance or a combination of the two. Cardiac output represents the amount of blood propelled into the circulation per unit of time. Total peripheral resistance is a calculated value and is estimated by the ratio of mean arterial pressure over cardiac output, expressed in arbitrary resistance units.

HEMODYNAMICS OF HYPERTENSION IN CHRONIC NONUREMIC, NONANEMIC RENAL PARENCHYMAL DISEASE

In contrast with essential hypertension, information regarding the hemodynamic changes of hypertension in early chronic renal parenchymal disease is limited.

Brod and associates[1] reported that cardiac output in patients with hypertension secondary to chronic nonuremic, nonanemic renal parenchymal disease was higher than in normotensive patients with renal parenchymal disease. Eleven of the 27 hypertensive patients had high cardiac output, and all 11 patients with high cardiac output had stage I-II hypertension as defined by the World Health Organization. None of the eight patients in stage III had high cardiac output. There was no difference in the total peripheral resistance between the normotensive renal patients and hypertensive renal patients with stage I-II hypertension. The total peripheral resistance in hypertensive renal patients with stage III hypertension was higher than that of patients with stage I-II. Therefore, Brod and coworkers postulated that hypertension secondary to renal parenchymal disease may be initiated by a high cardiac output, and at this stage total peripheral resistance is within normal range. The total peripheral resistance starts to increase only with the progress of hypertension to stage III, and this is the reason for the cardiac output decreasing again to its original level.

We have studied 23 patients with chronic renal parenchymal disease without uremia or anemia.[2] There were 15 males and 8 females ranging in age from 16 to 55 years, with a mean age of 36 years. Of the 23 patients studied, 9 were normotensive and showed no clinical, radiologic, or electrocardiographic changes of hypertensive cardiovascular disease or hypertensive retinopathy. Fourteen patients were hypertensive. Patients were excluded from this study if they had a documented family history of essential hypertension or were in the malignant phase of hypertension. Patients with a serum creatinine of 4 mg/dl or less and a hematocrit of 30 percent or more were included. Of the 9 normotensive patients, 5 had chronic glomerulonephritis, while polycystic kidney disease, diabetic glomerulosclerosis, chronic interstitial nephritis, and cystic disease in a solitary kidney each occurred in one patient. Of the 14 hypertensive patients, 9 had chronic glomerulonephritis, 4 had diabetic glomerulosclerosis, and 1 had multiple renal infarctions. The diagnoses were based on kidney biopsy, except for a patient with cystic renal disease where the diagnosis was confirmed by intravenous pyelogram and renal arteriography. The groups of hypertensive patients and normotensive patients were comparable for age, hematocrit, and inulin clearance. The systemic hemodynamics of hypertensive and normotensive patients with nonuremic renal parenchymal disease are shown in Figure 1. The average mean arterial pressure was 126 $\pm$ 3 mm Hg (mean $\pm$ S.E.) in hypertensive patients and 87 $\pm$ 3 mm Hg in normotensive patients ($p < 0.0005$) (Fig. 1A). The mean cardiac index in the hypertensive patients was 3.62 $\pm$ 0.20 liters/min/m^2 (mean $\pm$ S.E.), and in normotensive patients the mean cardiac index was 3.14 $\pm$ 0.1 liters/min/m^2 ($p < 0.05$) (Fig. 1B). The mean heart rate was 77 $\pm$ 3 beats/min in hypertensive patients and 66 $\pm$ 3 beats/min in normotensive patients ($p < 0.01$) (Fig. 1C). The mean stroke index in hypertensive patients was 47 $\pm$ 3 ml/stroke/m^2. In normotensive patients the mean stroke index was 47 $\pm$ 1 ml/stroke/m^2 (Fig. 1D). The

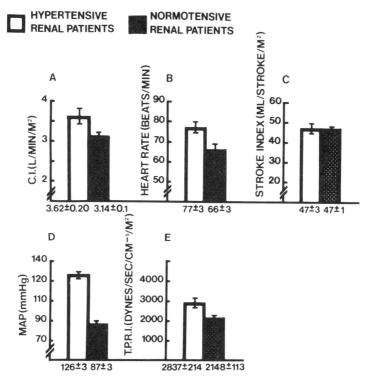

FIGURE 1. Comparisons of (A) cardiac index (C.I.), (B) heart rate, (C) stroke index, (D) mean arterial pressure (MAP), and (E) total peripheral resistance index (T.P.R.I.) of 14 hypertensive and 9 normotensive patients with chronic nonuremic renal parenchymal disease. Hemodynamic values are expressed as mean ± S.E. (From Kim, et al.,[2] with permission.)

mean total peripheral resistance index was 2837 ± 214 dynes/sec/cm^{-5}/m^2 in hypertensive patients and 2148 ± 113 dynes/sec/cm^{-5}/m^2 in normotensive patients ($p < 0.0125$) (Fig. 1E).

The patients with chronic renal parenchymal disease and hypertension were arbitrarily divided into those with hypertension of less than two years duration and those with disease of more than two years duration. The average mean arterial pressure was similar in the two subgroups (Fig. 2B). The mean cardiac index was higher in the patients with a more recent onset of hypertension (Fig. 2A), while the mean total peripheral resistance index was lower in this group (Fig. 2C).

This study shows that the overall cardiac index and heart rate of hypertensive patients with chronic renal parenchymal disease was higher than that of normotensive patients with chronic renal parenchymal disease. These findings suggest that in some patients the hypertension of nonuremic renal parenchymal disease is associated with a high cardiac output. When the hypertensive patients were divided into two subgroups according to the known duration of hypertension, it was suggested that the patients at an early stage of renal hypertension had a higher cardiac output. The pilot study suggests that with the progression of hypertension the cardiac output may decrease, while total peripheral resistance increases. This hemodynamic natural history is similar to the well documented natural history of essential hypertension.[3-11] However, more extensive studies of the hemodynamic changes of early stages of hypertension in chronic renal disease and of their possible evolution are necessary for a definite conclusion.

HEMODYNAMICS OF HYPERTENSION IN CHRONIC END-STAGE RENAL DISEASE

Hemodynamic Changes in Chronic End-Stage Renal Disease with Anemia

The hemodynamic pattern of hypertension in chronic end-stage renal disease is now well established.[15-18] The hemodynamic studies of 75 patients with end-stage renal disease (hypertensive and normotensive) are compared with those of 42 normal subjects in Figure 3.

The mean value of the hematocrit in normal subjects was 43 percent, while the uremic patients were all significantly anemic with a mean hematocrit of 23 percent.

In the 42 normal controls the mean cardiac index was 3.39 ± 0.08 L/min/m^2 (mean $\pm$ S.E.). In the 75 patients with end-stage renal disease the mean cardiac index was 4.44 ± 0.11 L/min/m^2 ($p < 0.001$) (Fig. 3A). The mean heart rate was 66 ± 1.2 beats/min in the 42 normal controls and 90 ± 1.1 beats/min in the 75 uremic patients ($p < 0.001$) (Fig. 3B). The 42 normal subjects had a mean stroke index of 52 ± 1.4 ml/stroke/m^2, and in the 75 uremic patients the mean stroke index was 50 ± 1.3 ml/stroke m^2 (Fig. 3C). The average mean arterial pressure in the 42 normal subjects was 91 ± 1.6 mm Hg., while in the 75 patients with end-stage renal disease the average mean arterial pressure was 125 ± 3.2 mm Hg. The difference is statistically significant ($p < 0.001$) and reflects the presence of hypertension in 52 of the 75 patients with end-stage renal disease (Fig. 3D). The calculated mean total peripheral resistance index was 2187 ± 59 dynes/sec/cm^{-5}/m^2 in the 42 normal subjects and 2389 ± 103 dynes/sec/cm^{-5}/m^2 in the 75 uremic patients. The difference is not statistically significant (Fig. 3E).

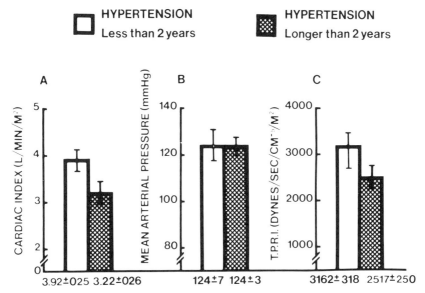

FIGURE 2. Comparisons of (A) cardiac index, (B) mean arterial pressure, and (C) total peripheral resistance index (T.P.R.I.) of 7 patients with chronic nonuremic renal parenchymal disease having hypertension of less than 2 years duration and 7 patients with chronic nonuremic renal parenchymal disease having hypertension of longer than 2 years duration. Hemodynamic values are expressed as mean ± S.E. (From Kim, et al.,[2] with permission.)

Hemodynamic Comparison Between Hypertensive and Normotensive Patients with End-Stage Renal Disease

Of the 75 patients studied, 23 were normotensive and 52 were hypertensive. The hemodynamic pattern of the 52 hypertensive patients was compared with that of the 23 normotensive patients. The results are shown in Figure 4.

The average mean arterial pressure in the 52 hypertensive uremic patients was 139 ± 2.9 mm Hg, while in the 23 normotensive uremic patients the average mean arterial pressure was 93 ± 1.8 mm Hg (p < 0.001) (Fig. 4A). The mean cardiac index in the 52 hypertensive uremic patients was 4.39 ± 0.14 L/min/m² and in the 23 normotensive uremic patients 4.55 ± 0.15 L/min/m². The difference is not significant (Fig. 4B). The mean heart rate was 91 ± 1.4 beats/min in the 52 hypertensive patients and 89 ± 2.0 beats/min in the 23 normotensive patients. The 52 hypertensive patients had a mean stroke index of 49 ± 1.6 ml/stroke/m²; the mean stroke index in the 23 normotensive patients was 51 ± 1.6 ml/stroke/m².

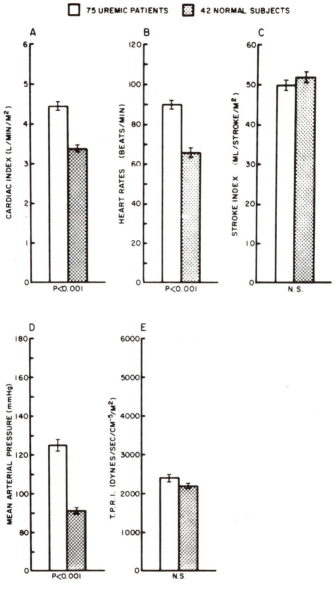

FIGURE 3. Cardiac index (A), heart rate (B), stroke index (C), mean arterial pressure (D), and total peripheral resistance index (T.P.R.I.) (E) of 75 patients with end-stage renal disease (hypertensive and normotensive, mean hematocrit 23 percent) compared with 42 normal controls (mean hematocrit 43 percent). Hemodynamic values are expressed as mean ± S.E. N.S. = not statistically significant. (From Kim, et al.,[15] with the permission of the American Heart Association, Inc.)

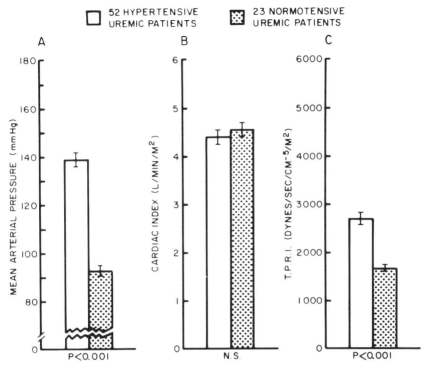

FIGURE 4. Comparison of (A) mean arterial pressure, (B) cardiac index, and (C) total peripheral resistance index (T.P.R.I.) of 52 hypertensive patients (mean hematocrit 23 percent) and 23 normotensive patients (mean hematocrit also 23 percent) with end-stage renal disease. (From Kim, et al.,[15] with the permission of the American Heart Association, Inc.)

Neither of these differences was significant. The calculated mean total peripheral resistance index was 2703 ± 120 dynes/sec/cm^{-5}/m^2 in the hypertensive patients and 1670 ± 61 dynes/sec/cm^{-5}/m^2 in the normotensive patients ($p < 0.001$) (Fig. 4C). The mean hematocrit was 23 percent in both the hypertensive and normotensive uremic patients. Therefore, the hypertension of chronic end-stage renal disease is sustained by an elevated total peripheral resistance.

Hemodynamic Effects of Correction of Anemia

Six of the 75 patients with end-stage renal disease underwent further study to test the effect of increasing the hematocrit. Hemodynamic studies were performed twice a week prior to hemodialysis at least 48 hours after the patient had received packed red cell transfusions during the previous hemodialysis. Blood was administered during hemodialysis as buffy-coat-free packed red cells. Hematocrit was increased to at least 40 percent in each patient. Body weight was maintained within 1.8 kg in each patient during the entire study period.

Serial transfusions of buffy-coat-free packed red cells resulted in a linear decrease in cardiac index to a normal level. The diastolic pressure increased as hematocrit increased. The total peripheral resistance index increased markedly as hematocrit increased. Neither body weight nor blood volume changed significantly during the study. The effect of increase in hematocrit on cardiac index, total peripheral resistance index, and mean arterial pressure in a representative patient is shown in Figure 5. With the increase in hematocrit there was a progressive decrease in cardiac index. The total peripheral resistance index and mean arterial pressure increased progressively as hematocrit increased. The most likely explanation for the increasing total peripheral resistance and the decreasing of cardiac output as a result of correcting the anemia is related to the oxygen delivery and the viscosity of the blood. Severe anemia is associated with inadequate oxygen delivery to the tissue. This condition produces peripheral vasodilatation. The hypoxic vasodilatation decreases the total peripheral resistance, and a decrease in the resistance to venous return which increases venous return and cardiac output. Anemia also decreases the viscosity of the blood, which decreases resistance to venous return and increases venous return and cardiac output.[19-21] Correcting the anemia abolishes hypoxic dilatation and increases the viscosity of the blood, which increases the peripheral resistance and blood pressure and decreases the venous return and cardiac output. This effect is probably magnified in previously hypertensive uremic patients.

Hemodynamic studies were performed in 11 patients before and after a successful renal transplantation. The mean hematocrit of the 11 patients before the renal transplantation was 20.9 percent and after a successful renal transplantation was 35.2 percent. With the increase in hematocrit after the renal transplantation, the mean cardiac index decreased from 4.58 L/min/m^2 to 3.78 L/min/m^2.

These studies indicated that the major factor responsible for high cardiac output in patients with chronic end-stage renal disease is anemia itself.

Duke and Abelmann[22] found cardiac index values of 4.73 L/min/m^2 and low total peripheral resistance in anemic patients with normal kidney function (a mean hematocrit of 20.3 percent). The hemodynamic pattern of their anemic patients and the degree of their anemia are very similar to those of the normotensive uremic patients in our study. In their study, the correction of anemia in the same patients resulted in a decrease of

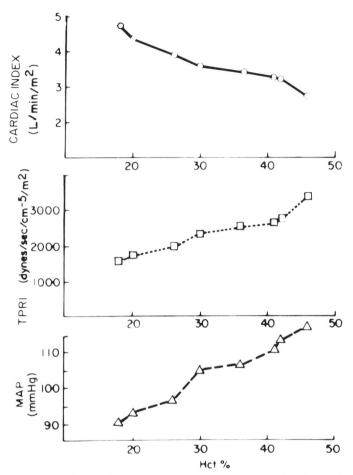

FIGURE 5. The effects of increase in hematocrit on cardiac index (o), total peripheral resistance (TPRI) (□) and mean arterial pressure (MAP) (△), in one particular patient. (From Kim, et al.,[17] with permission.)

cardiac index to normal (3.44 L/min/m²) and a significant increase in total peripheral resistance.

Hemodynamic Effects of Bilateral Nephrectomy

The hemodynamic studies in 12 patients with chronic end-stage renal disease and severe but nonmalignant hypertension who underwent bilateral nephrectomy are shown in Figure 6. The hemodynamic studies are compared at equivalent levels of total exchangeable sodium and body weight for each patient before and after bilateral nephrectomy.

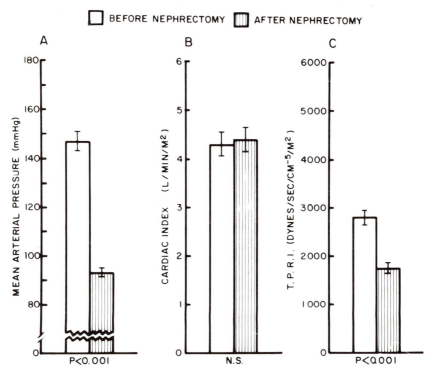

FIGURE 6. Mean arterial pressure (A), cardiac index (B), and total peripheral resistance index (T.P.R.I.) (C) before and after bilateral nephrectomy in 12 hypertensive patients (severe but nonmalignant) with end-stage renal disease. The hemodynamic values of each patient are compared at equivalent levels of exchangeable sodium and body weight. Exchangeable sodium ranged from 42 to 47 mEq/kg before nephrectomy and 41 to 49 mEq/kg after nephrectomy, indicating these patients were studied at dry weight. (From Kim, et al.,[15] with the permission of the American Heart Association, Inc.)

Bilateral nephrectomy resulted in a significant reduction of blood pressure in all 12 patients. The average mean arterial pressure decreased from 147 mm Hg to 93 mm Hg (p < 0.001) (Fig. 6A). Changes in cardiac index (Fig. 6B), heart rate, and stroke index were not statistically significant. As a consequence, a reduction in total peripheral resistance index occurred after bilateral nephrectomy in every case, from a mean of 2804 dynes/sec/cm^{-5}/m^2 to a mean of 1746 dynes/sec/cm^{-5}/m^2 (p < 0.001) (Fig. 6C).

Bilateral nephrectomy was performed in an additional group of 8 patients with chronic end-stage renal disease and hypertension in the malignant phase. Removal of both kidneys resulted in a dramatic decrease of blood pressure in every case. The average mean arterial pressure decreased from 158 mm Hg to 112 mm Hg (p < 0.001) (Fig. 7A). In contrast to the group of patients with nonmalignant hypertension in whom the cardiac index was not changed by bilateral nephrectomy, cardiac index increased after bilateral nephrectomy in each case of malignant hypertension. The mean cardiac index was 3.45 L/min/m^2 before bilateral nephrectomy and rose to 4.40 L/min/m^2 after bilateral nephrectomy (p < 0.001) (Fig. 7B). Changes in heart rate were minor and inconsistent, while the stroke index increased after nephrectomy in every case. The mean stroke index was 38 ml/stroke/m^2 before bilateral nephrectomy and became 51 ml/stroke/m^2 after bilateral nephrectomy (p < 0.001) (Fig. 7C). For equivalent levels of total exchangeable sodium, the total peripheral resistance index was invariably lower in the absence of renal tissue (Fig. 7D).

The difference in hemodynamic patterns in malignant and nonmalignant renal hypertension warrants some comments. Cardiac output and stroke index are lower in the malignant hypertension group, and peripheral resistance is higher. A similar hemodynamic pattern of low cardiac output and high total peripheral resistance has been described in experimental malignant hypertension.[23-25] The hemodynamic differences observed in our patients, as well as those reported in the experimental animal,[23-25] suggest a qualitatively different vasopressor mechanism in malignant hypertension.

Bilateral nephrectomy was performed in 8 normotensive patients with end-stage renal disease. The hemodynamic studies were compared for each patient at the same body weight before and after bilateral nephrectomy. Bilateral nephrectomy resulted in no significant change in mean arterial pressure, cardiac index, and total peripheral resistance index.

In summary, patients with end-stage renal disease had significantly higher cardiac indexes than did normal controls, while stroke indexes were not different from those of normals. The higher cardiac indexes of uremic patients were accounted for by increased heart rates. Cardiac index, heart rate, and stroke index were the same in hypertensive and normotensive uremic patients, while mean total peripheral resistance indices of hypertensive uremic patients were higher than in normotensive uremic patients. Therefore, the hypertension in end-stage renal disease is sustained by a high total peripheral resistance.

The serial hemodynamic studies during the correction of anemia and hemodynamic studies before and after a successful renal transplantation indicate that the major factor responsible for high cardiac output in patients with end-stage renal disease is anemia itself.

The hemodynamic studies before and after bilateral nephrectomy in the 12 severe but nonmalignant hypertensive uremic patients and the 8 uremic patients with malignant hypertension showed a marked reduction

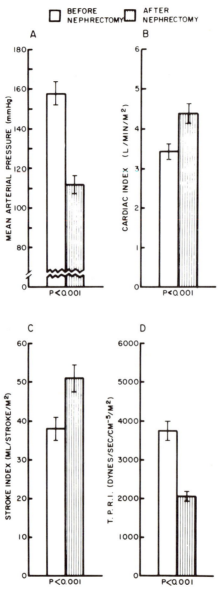

FIGURE 7. Mean arterial pressure (A), cardiac index (B), stroke index (C), and total peripheral resistance index (T.P.R.I.) (D) before and after bilateral nephrectomy in 8 patients with end-stage renal disease and malignant hypertension. Hemodynamic values of each patient are compared at an equivalent level of total exchangeable sodium and body weight. Exchangeable sodium ranged from 43 to 49 mEq/kg before nephrectomy and 45 to 48 mEq/kg after nephrectomy. (From Kim, et al.,[15] with the permission of the American Heart Association, Inc.)

of blood pressure after bilateral nephrectomy. This reduction of blood pressure after bilateral nephrectomy was due to a decrease in total peripheral resistance.

These findings imply that a vasopressor substance or substances of renal origin increasing peripheral resistance is the major factor in the pathophysiology of severe and malignant hypertension in end-stage renal disease.

Bilateral nephrectomy in normotensive uremic patients resulted in no significant change in mean arterial pressure, cardiac index, and total peripheral resistance index.

REGULATION OF BLOOD PRESSURE IN END-STAGE RENAL DISEASE AND THE ANEPHRIC STATE

Hypertension in anephric patients and those with end-stage kidney failure is sustained by a high total peripheral resistance.[15,26] The most important factors responsible for the increase in total peripheral resistance in patients with end-stage kidneys are the vasopressor function of the kidney[15,26] and an increase in body salt and water.[26-29] In anephric patients, salt and water balance plays a major role in the regulation of blood pressure.[26,29-33] The final effect of salt and water loading in the anephric patient has been found to be an increase in total peripheral resistance.[26,33] The precise mechanism, however, by which expansion of body fluid increases blood pressure is not known.[26,33]

Anephric patients and those with end-stage kidneys on maintenance hemodialysis have no renal excretory function, and their body fluids are controlled by their salt and fluid intake and by the amount of salt and water removed by the artificial kidney. Therefore, patients' body weights can be controlled by varying these parameters.

Coleman and coworkers[33] reported their sequential hemodynamic studies during volume expansion in three anephric patients. They showed that the increase in blood pressure during volume expansion was associated with an initial increase in cardiac output followed by an increase in total peripheral resistance. It has been postulated that the initial increase in cardiac output results in perfusion of the peripheral tissues above their metabolic needs. This would elicit myogenic constriction of peripheral vessels with consequent increase in total peripheral resistance[33-35] (theory of whole-body autoregulation).

We[29,36] performed sequential hemodynamic studies during volume expansion in 4 anephric patients and 6 patients with end-stage kidneys. This study resulted in four different sequential hemodynamic patterns: 1) no significant increase in blood pressure in 2 patients; 2) increase in blood pressure associated with an increase in cardiac output and without change in total peripheral resistance in 2 patients; 3) increase in blood pressure associated with an increase in total peripheral resistance from the beginning without an increase in cardiac output in 5 patients; 4) increase in blood pressure associated with an initial increase in cardiac output followed by an increase in total peripheral resistance in 1 patient.

This study indicates that an initial increase in cardiac output is not necessary to increase blood pressure during salt and water loading in either anephric patients or those with end-stage kidneys. Furthermore, a sustained increase in cardiac output during salt and water loading is not always followed by an increase in total peripheral resistance. Mechanisms other than whole-body autoregulation play a role in increasing blood pressure during salt and water loading in patients deprived of renal excretory function.

The pharmacokinetics of drugs used in the management of cardiovascular disease with specific reference to antihypertensive agents is discussed in Chapter 3. The rationale for their use is elaborated on in Chapter 9.

REFERENCES

1. Brod, J., Cachovan, M., Bahlman, N.J., et al.: Haemodynamic basis of hypertension, in chronic non-uraemic parenchymatous renal disease, in Giovannetti, S., Bonomini, V., D'Amico, G. (eds.): Proceedings 6th International Congress of Nephrology. S. Karger, Basel, 1976, p. 305.
2. Kim, K.E., Onesti, G., Fernandes, M., et al.: Hemodynamics of hypertension, in Onesti, G., Fernandes, M., Kim, K.E. (eds.): Regulation of Blood Pressure by the Central Nervous System. Grune & Stratton, New York, 1976, p. 337.
3. Eich, R.H., Peters, R.J., Cuddy, R.P., et al.: The hemodynamics in labile hypertension. Am. Heart J. 63:188, 1962.
4. Finkielman, S., Worcel, M., and Agrest, A.: Hemodynamic pattern in essential hypertension. Circulation 31:356, 1965.
5. Bello, C.T., Sevy, R.W., and Harakal, C.: Varying hemodynamic patterns in essential hypertension. Am. J. Med. Sci. 250:24, 1965.
6. Eich, R., Cuddy, R.P., Smulyan, H., et al.: Hemodynamics in labile hypertension: follow-up study. Circulation 34:299, 1966.
7. Sannerstedt, R.: Hemodynamic response to exercise in patients with arterial hypertension. Acta Med. Scand. 180 (Suppl. 458):1, 1966.
8. Lund-Johansen, P.: Hemodynamics in early essential hypertension. Acta Med. Scand. 181 (Suppl. 482):1, 1967.
9. Frohlich, E.D., Tarazi, R.C., and Dustan, H.P.: Reexamination of the hemodynamics of hypertension. Am. J. Med. Sci. 257:9, 1969.
10. Nestel, P.J.: Blood pressure and catecholamine excretion after mental stress in labile hypertension. Lancet 1:692, 1969.
11. Safar, M.E., Fendler, J-P., Weil, B., et al.: Etude hemodynamique de l'hypertension arterielle labile. Presse Med. 78:111, 1970.
12. Julius, S., Pascual, A.V., Sannerstedt, R., et al.: Relationship between cardiac

output and peripheral resistance in borderline hypertension. Circulation, 43:382, 1971.

13. Julius, S., Pascual, A.V., and London, R.: Role of parasympathetic inhibition in the hyperkinetic type of borderline hypertension. Circulation 46:413, 1971.

14. Lund-Johansen, P.: Hemodynamic trends in untreated essential hypertension. Preliminary report on a 10 year follow-up study. Acta Med. Scand. (Suppl. 602):68, 1976.

15. Kim, K.E., Onesti, G., Schwartz, A.B., et al.: Hemodynamics of hypertension in chronic end-stage renal disease. Circulation, 46:456, 1972.

16. Neff, M.S., Kim, K.E., Persoff, M., et al.: Hemodynamics of uremic anemia. Circulation 43:876, 1971.

17. Kim, K.E., Onesti, G., Neff, M.D., et al.: Hemodynamic alterations in hypertension of chronic end-stage renal disease, in Onesti, G., Kim, K.E., Moyer, J.H. (eds.): Hypertension: Mechanisms and Management. Grune & Stratton, New York, 1973, p. 609.

18. Kim, K.E., Onesti, G., and Swartz, C.D.: Hemodynamics of hypertension in uremia. Kidney Int. 7 (Suppl. 2):155, 1975.

19. Whittaker, S.R.F., and Winton, F.R.: The apparent viscosity of blood flowing in the isolated hindlimb of the dog, and its variation with corpuscular concentration. J. Physiol. (Lond.) 78:339, 1933.

20. Guyton, A.C., and Richardson, T.Q.: Effect of hematocrit on venous return. Circ. Res. 9:157, 1961.

21. Guyton, A.C., Jones, C.E., and Coleman, T.G.: Circulatory Physiology: Cardiac Output and Its Regulation. W.B. Saunders, Philadelphia, 1973, p. 396.

22. Duke, M., and Abelmann, W.H.: The hemodynamic response to chronic anemia. Circulation 39:503, 1969.

23. Ledingham, J.M., and Pelling, D.: Cardiac output and peripheral resistance in experimental renal hypertension. Circ. Res. 20–21 (Suppl. II):187, 1967.

24. Ferrario, C.M., Page, I.H., and McCubbin, J.W.: Increased cardiac output as a contributory factor in experimental renal hypertension in dogs. Circ. Res. 27:799, 1970.

25. Ferrario, C.M.: Contribution of cardiac output and peripheral resistance to experimental renal hypertension. Am. J. Physiol. 226:711, 1974.

26. Onesti, G., Kim, K.E., Greco, J.A., et al.: Blood pressure regulation in end-stage renal disease and anephric man. Circ. Res. 26 (Suppl. I):145, 1975.

27. Vertes, V., Cangiano, J.L., and Berman, L.B.: Hypertension in end-stage renal disease. N. Engl. J. Med., 280:978, 1969.

28. Weidmann, P., Maxwell, M.N., and Lupa, A.N.: Plasma renin activity and blood pressure in terminal renal failure. N. Engl. J. Med. 285:757, 1971.

29. Kim, K.E., Onesti, G., DelGuercio, E.T., et al.: Sequential hemodynamic changes in end-stage renal disease and the anephric state during volume expansion. Hypertension 2:102, 1980.

30. Dustan, H.P., and Page, I.N.: Some factors in renal and renoprival hypertension. J. Lab. Clin. Med., 64:948, 1964.

31. Merrill, J.P., Giodano, C., and Heetderks, D.R.: Role of the kidney in human hypertension: 1. Failure of hypertension to develop in the renoprival subject. Am. J. Med. 31:391, 1961.

32. DelGreco, F., and Burgess, J.L.: Hypertension in terminal renal failure: Observations pre and post bilateral nephrectomy. J. Chronic Dis. 26:471, 1973.

33.   Coleman, T.G., Bower, J.D., Langford, N.G., et al.: Regulation of arterial pressure in the anephric state. Circulation, 42:509, 1970.
34.   Coleman, T.G., Granger, H.J., and Guyton, A.C.: Whole body circulatory autoregulation and hypertension. Circ. Res. 28 and 29 (Suppl. 2):76, 1971.
35.   Ledingham, J.M.: Blood pressure regulation in renal failure. J.R. Coll. Physicians. 5:103, 1971.
36.   Kim, K.E., Onesti, G., DelGuercio, E.T., et al.: The hemodynamic response to salt and water loading in patient with end-stage renal disease and anephric man. Clin. Sci. Mol. Med. 51 (Suppl. 3):223, 1976.

3

CLINICAL PHARMACOLOGY OF CARDIOVASCULAR DRUGS

DAVID T. LOWENTHAL, M.D., AND MELTON B. AFFRIME, PHARM. D.

BIOTRANSFORMATION

Drugs given to patients with renal failure undergo the conventional processes of biotransformation: absorption, distribution, metabolism, and elimination (A, D, M, E). However, abnormalities in these processes make the azotemic patient predisposed to adverse drug reactions (ADR). Smith and coworkers[1] found that the incidence of adverse drug reactions was greater on a medical service when the patients' serum urea nitrogen was greater than 40 mg/dl. Although this was a crude way at the time of assessing renal function, it opened the horizons to clinical research in which one could elucidate the causes for such adverse drug reactions. It is now appreciated that the causes of drug toxicity in renal failure[2] are impaired renal excretion of parent drug or active metabolite(s), altered hepatic metabolism (increased or decreased), increased sensitivity (alteration in target organ response) due to altered protein binding, abnormal blood brain barrier, and drug interactions, both pharmacokinetic (A, D, M, E) and pharmacodynamic (blood pressure, pulse, and so forth).

An understanding of the ways these patients differ from normal can enable one to individualize therapy for this group of people and to achieve better therapeutic results. Specifically, cardiovascular disease occurs in high frequency in end-stage renal disease,[3] the complications of which may be related to hypertension or irregularities in rate and rhythm. Thus, it has been necessary to devise studies to obtain information regarding the biotransformation of commonly used antiarrhythmic drugs, digitalis, and antihypertensive agents.

Absorption

In general, the absorption of cardiovascular drugs is unimpaired in patients with renal failure. Anderson and coworkers[4] have suggested that gastric absorption is affected by an increase in salivary urea and gastric ammonia, but clinical situations have not corroborated any problems with drug absorption.

Drug Distribution

Drug distribution may influence the time of onset, the magnitude, and the duration of drug action. Distribution can be modified by physiologic factors and disease states since it depends on regional tissue blood flow, cardiac output, pH gradient, plasma protein binding, and the permeability of cell membranes to unionized drugs. However, from a practical point of view, in renal failure, abnormalities of drug distribution are important for two main reasons:[5,6] 1) concentration of active drug at receptors may be changed, i.e., altered protein binding and 2) the rate of drug elimination may be decreased in patients with chronic renal failure since elimination depends on the volume of distribution. A decrease in the volume of distribution of certain drugs may be due to diminished muscle mass, decreased red blood cell mass (anemia), and anatomic absence of renal tissue.

Plasma Drug-Protein Binding in Uremia

Proposals to individualize drug dosages to achieve a "therapeutic" plasma level assume knowledge of the "therapeutic" concentration. For a number of drugs, such information exists.[7] This information, however, has nearly always been obtained in patients without renal failure. Under certain circumstances, plasma concentrations of drugs that are thought to be therapeutic in normal persons will be toxic in azotemic or uremic patients. These circumstances occur when an acidic organic drug is normally highly protein bound but whose binding is decreased by renal failure. The organic acid anticonvulsant phenytoin (Dilantin) is such a drug. Organic bases, in general, have normal protein binding.

The intensity of a drug's effect is related to its concentration in plasma water since it is this concentration that sets the diffusion gradient for the drug to the site of action. All of the analytical methods for drugs measure both drug in plasma water and drug bound to plasma protein. For this reason, the relationship between the total drug concentration in plasma and the intensity of effect will only be good if there are no changes in the protein binding of the drug. If protein binding of the drug is constant, then drug concentration in plasma water will be proportional to the total drug concentration and one can relate either to the intensity of effect. If, on the other hand, protein binding of the drug is decreased, such as occurs with phenytoin or other organic acids in renal failure, then these relationships will change and the intensity of effect will be greater than expected for any particular total drug concentration in plasma. Under these conditions, as azotemia progresses one should decrease the values used for "therapeutic" plasma concentrations to allow for this decreased protein binding.[8]

Drugs Metabolized to Inactive Compounds

The effect of renal failure on the apparent elimination rate of cardiovascular drugs studied in man is presented in Table 1. Most drugs that are metabolized by microsomal oxidations have normal or accelerated elimination rates in patients with chronic renal failure.[9]

The accelerated metabolism of phenytoin is of major importance in individualizing dosage of this drug for patients with seizures in chronic renal failure. Average values for phenytoin half-life in control and uremic subjects are shown in Table 2. Thus, uremic patients require, on the average, 100 to 400 mg phenytoin daily to achieve the usual therapeutic concentrations in plasma water.[11,12] This high concentration of phenytoin may not be needed for seizure control in all azotemic patients, however, since in progressive renal failure uremic patients have been reported as having seizure control with the lower plasma levels achieved by the customary doses of phenytoin.[9,12,13]

Drug Metabolite Accumulation Renal Failure

While traditionally one thinks of drug biotransformation pathways as inactivating or detoxification pathways, this is not necessarily the case. Some drug metabolites are pharmacologically active, accumulate in renal failure, and cause effects not necessarily observed in patients with healthy kidneys. An example of this is meperidine (Demerol).

Meperidine is normally metabolized to normeperidine that may then be either excreted in the urine or further metabolized. Normeperidine has been shown in animals to have less analgesic potency but more convulsant potency than meperidine. Patients with renal failure given meperidine for post-transplantation analgesia have marked accumulation of normeperidine after a few doses of the parent drug. It has been shown that in patients with poor renal function receiving meperidine and having signs and symptoms of central nervous system irritability including seizures, high normeperidine levels existed. The meperidine was

TABLE 1. Effect of renal failure on elimination rate of cardiovascular drugs. (This is only a guideline. Individual plasma concentration must be correlated with therapeutic effect for ideal monitoring.)

Drug	Half-life ($T^{1/2}$) in:		% Excreted in urine unchanged	Extra-renal elimination	Plasma protein binding (%, NRF)	Dosage interval (hr) with C creat of:				Dialyzability
	NRF (hr)	ESRD (hr)				≥80 ml/min	50–79 ml/min	30–49 ml/min	<30 ml/min	
Antihypertensive agents										
Clonidine	4–24	48	30–47 (Avg. 50%)	H	20–40%	12	12	12	12	HD slow
Diazoxide	21–36	>30	100	N	90–93*	Rapid bolus determined by response				PD
Guanethidine	3–4	48–70	25–50	H		24	24	AVOID		?
Hydralazine	2–8	2–8		HG	87	8	8	8	8–16	PD
Methyldopa	8–20	5	20–55	H	20	6	6	9–12	12–24	PD
Metoprolol	3–4	?	3	H	11	8	8	8	8	
Minoxidil	2–5	2–4	1	H						
Nitroprusside	0.1	0.1	1	H		constant IV infusion				Thiocyanate PD
Reserpine	46–168	45–323	1	H		24	24	AVOID		
Prazosin	2.5–4	1.8–4.5	2–4	H	97†	8–12	8–12	6–12	8–12	
Propranolol	2–6	4.4	5	H	90–96†	6–12	6–12	6–12	6–12	
Timolol	4	4	20	H	10	12	12	12	AVOID	HD
Cardiac glycosides										
Digitoxin	72–200	120–200	8–30	H	90–97*	24	24	24	24–36	PD slow
Digoxin	30–40	87–110	95	G	2–3	24	24–36	36–48	48–72	PD slow
Ouabain	14–20	60–70	37–50	H		12–24	24	24–36	36–48	PD slow

Diuretics

	t½ NRF	t½ ESRD	% Excreted	Route	% Protein bound		Dose interval (hr)			HD
Amiloride	6–10	N.A.	50	H	90–95	12–24	24		AVOID	
Chlorathiazide	2	4–6	100	H	20–80	12	12		AVOID	
Ethacrynic Acid	0.5–1	10	20	H		24	24		AVOID	
Furosemide	3–5		67	H	90–97*	NO CHANGE				HD
Hydrochloro-thiazide	4	4–6	45–62			12–24	12–24		AVOID	
Metolazone	4	?		H	98	24	24		AVOID	
Spironolactone	13–24	N.A.		H	67*	6	6		AVOID	
Triamterene	2	N.A.				12	12		AVOID	

Antiarrhythmics

	t½ NRF	t½ ESRD	% Excreted	Route	% Protein bound		Dose interval (hr)			HD
Disopyramide	4.4–8.2	43	50–60	H	60	6	6	6–8	12–24	HD
Lidocaine	0.75–2	0.75–2	2–3	H	60–65	IV INFUSION				
Phenytoin	10–16	6–10	65	H	89–91*	8–24	8–24	8–24		HD slow
Procainamide	2.2–4	9–16	45–65	H	15	3	3	4–6	AVOID	HD
Quinidine	3–16	3–16	10–50	H	80	6–12	6–12	6–12	6–12	HD
Bretylium 133	8.1	31.5	80			Individualized based upon response				

Abbr.: NRF = normal renal function; ESRD = end-stage renal failure; H = hepatic; G = gastrointestinal; N = nonrenal (precise route unknown); C creat = creatinine clearance; HD = hemodialysis; PD = peritoneal dialysis; N.A. = not applicable.
*Decreased binding in abnormal renal function.
†No change in binding in abnormal renal function.

TABLE 2. Average values for phenytoin half-life

Study	Half-Life (hours)	
	Control	Uremic
Letteri[10]	13 ± 0.2	8 ± 2
Odar-Cederlof[11]	13 ± 2	8 ± 2

stopped, and the central nervous system irritability subsided. This decline in CNS irritability seemed to parallel the fall of normeperidine levels in the one patient in whom it was measured.[14]

Thus, it appears that normeperidine can accumulate in patients with renal failure given multiple doses of meperidine. This high level of normeperidine can cause CNS excitation. In contrast, morphine is metabolized to morphine glucuronide, a metabolite that is unlikely to have very much effect on the central nervous system. Hence, it would appear that patients with renal failure who require frequent narcotic doses for more than several days are less likely to have CNS excitation as a side effect if they are given morphine instead of meperidine.

Procainamide is excreted unchanged or acetylated to N-acetylprocainamide which is then eliminated from the body by urinary excretion. N-acetylprocainamide has an action on the heart that is similar to procainamide. Patients with renal failure receiving procainamide at dosages approximately reduced to correct for the slower than normal elimination of procainamide still had marked accumulation of N-acetylprocainamide. The intensity of effect observed, both therapeutic and toxic, was clearly related to this metabolite accumulation as well as the procainamide itself.[15]

Other drugs with active metabolites that accumulate in renal failure include chlorophenyoxyisobutyric acid, the free-acid active metabolite of clofibrate, and oxypurinol, an active metabolite of allopurinol.[16,17]

Drug Elimination—Drugs Excreted Unchanged

Drug excretion (renal, biliary) is only one facet of drug elimination. By definition, once the liver has transformed the parent drug into an active or inactive metabolite the parent compound has been "eliminated."

A relatively small number of drugs are eliminated from the body by renal excretion of the drug itself. Digoxin, aminoglycosides, and furosemide are examples of drugs excreted unchanged. Methods for reducing the usual doses of these drugs for patients with renal failure have been published [2,18-21] and are now standard practice. All of the methods proposed involve reducing the daily dose of the drug in proportion to the degree of reduction of renal function. This dosage reduction can be accomplished by either reducing the usual dose and keeping the usual dosing interval unchanged, prolonging the dosing interval and keeping the usual dose unchanged, or a combination of lowering the dose and prolonging the dosing intervals. This last method is the one most frequently chosen.

The elimination of pharmacologic agents that are excreted largely unchanged in the urine is best described by the drug half-life ($T^{1}/_{2}$), that is, the time in which plasma concentration falls to one-half the peak level. Half-life is related to the renal clearance and apparent volume of distribution within body water[22] by the equation $T^{1}/_{2} = 0.693 \times$ volume of distribution of the drug divided by renal clearance; where $T^{1}/_{2}$ is in minutes, 0.693 is the natural logarithm of 2, and the renal clearance is in ml/min. The half-life, therefore, varies directly with the apparent volume of distribution and inversely with the renal clearance. Profound alterations of pharmacologic affect may occur by modifications of either of these factors.

While one can always show a good average correlation between the elimination rate of the drug and the amount of renal function present, there is large individual variation about the average. Any individual patient may have faster or slower drug elimination than average. Thus, the dosage calculated by any of the standard ways,[2,18-21] no matter how precise the calculation, must be considered a rough estimate of the proper dose and not assumed to be the patient's correct dose. This estimated starting dose can then be individualized for the particular patient in the usual way of adjusting it in accordance with the intensity of effect or response produced in the patient, or the dose can be adjusted to achieve a desired concentration of drug in the patient's blood plasma or serum.

The pharmacokinetics of the cardiovascular drugs which have been studied in patients with renal insufficiency will each be reviewed separately.

DIGITALIS PREPARATIONS

Digoxin and digitoxin are the two most commonly used digitalis glycosides today. They find wide clinical usage for both their inotropic and antiarrhythmic effects. However, wide usage has been accompanied by widespread toxicity. Up to 23 percent of inpatients receiving digoxin have evidence of digitalis toxicity.[23,24] Even more significantly, these digitalis toxic patients had twice the mortality of nontoxic patients. Familiarity with the details of the clinical pharmacology and pharmacokinetics of these two glycosides, especially as they compare and contrast to each other, is necessary to avoid untoward effects. Indeed, a decrease in the incidence of digitalis toxicity has been noted when glycoside therapy is guided by appropriate pharmacokinetic models and digitalis plasma concentration measurements[25-27] (see Table 1).

Pharmacokinetics and Plasma Protein Binding Digoxin and Digitoxin in Renal Disease

From the known clinical pharmacology of digoxin and digitoxin in normal persons, it can be predicted that since digoxin is more dependent on renal excretion, its elimination will be significantly hindered in patients with renal failure. In general, digoxin clearance parallels and decreases as creatinine clearance is impaired.[28-30] As renal impairment progresses there is an increase in the fecal excretion of digoxin.[29] However, this alternate pathway of digoxin elimination cannot completely compensate for the loss of the renal excretory route and overall elimination of digoxin is impaired.[31-33] Digoxin half-life can be prolonged as much as 4 to 10 days in patients with renal failure.[34] Nonetheless, no significant change in digoxin dosage is advised until the creatinine clearance is less than 50 ml/min, i.e., no change is needed for patients undergoing unilateral nephrectomy.[35] A decrease in digoxin dose of 50 percent with a creatinine of 3 to 5 mg percent and a decrease in digoxin dose of 75 percent in patients without renal function is advised.[28,30,36] Nomogram methods most commonly use serum creatinine to judge digoxin dosage.[37]

Recently, the formula used to assess digoxin dosage in uremic patients based on creatinine alone has been challenged along several lines. The correlation of digoxin half-life and creatinine clearance was shown to be poor ($r = 0.4$).[38] Furthermore, the volume of distribution of digoxin is both decreased[39] and very variable in patients with renal failure. Thus, digoxin clearance as predicted from serum creatinine alone does not predict digoxin half-life in a simple fashion.[40,41] Others, citing that digoxin is handled by tubular as well as glomerular mechanisms, suggest that the blood urea nitrogen concentration might better be used to adjust digoxin dosage.[42] This has not found wide clinical application. Still others suggest measuring digoxin urinary output to circumvent the problem of variability in digoxin volume of distribution.[43] Digoxin clearance (ml/min) may be calculated by obtaining a timed urinary digoxin concentration (mg/min) and drawing a digoxin serum level (ng/ml) at the mid-point of the urinary collection. Six nomogram methods for calculating digoxin doses in renal failure have been compared in the literature.[43]

As a general rule, serum digoxin half-life in patients with severe renal failure can be estimated to be four days.[28,44,45] This means that 14 percent of the digoxin in the body is excreted by nonurinary routes per day and that 14 percent is necessary to maintain steady state total body stores. Of interest is the fact that if one neglects to discontinue digoxin for 2 days with concurrent absolute decrease in renal function for 2 days, there is only a 21 percent increase in total body digoxin stores. Thus, although renal function is of great clinical importance in judging digoxin dosage, it is frequently not as critical as may be thought.[32]

Although it has been stated that only the maintenance dose of digoxin needs to be changed in patients with uremia,[45] the decrease in volume of distribution of digoxin in uremic patients suggests that a decrease in initial dosage may be warranted in some cases. In addition, the binding of digoxin to serum proteins was shown to be significantly decreased in the face of uremia (25 $\pm$ 4 percent in controls vs. 18 $\pm$ 6 percent in uremic plasma, p <0.01).[46] However, such a change amounts to only a 10 percent increase in the free fraction of digoxin and is usually not of clinical importance.

There is some disagreement about the effect of uremia on digitoxin metabolism, binding, and excretion. Some authors[47] have reasoned that although renal elimination of digitoxin is a minor pathway of bioelimination and amounts to only 30 percent of drug elimination in normal persons that this is sufficient to cause alterations in digitoxin pharmacokinetics in uremic patients. It has been estimated that uremic patients eliminate only 7.6 percent of their digitoxin stores per day as opposed to the normal 11 percent elimination per day. This would result in a prolongation of digitoxin half-life to 8.77 days. Thus, a formula for digitoxin maintenance dosage is 7.7 + (0.035 $\times$ creatinine clearance) mg.

The pharmacokinetics of digitoxin in uremic patients is more complex than this but the net result is that little alteration in digitoxin dosage is necessary. Digitoxin binding may be decreased in uremic patients because in general they have lower plasma protein levels. In addition, there seems to be a shift in the metabolites of digitoxin to cardioactive metabolites with lower affinity for protein binding sites. Therefore, in uremic patients with decreased plasma proteins, serum concentrations of digitoxin tend to be lower but the total active unbound drug concentration is near normal.[46,48,49] Furthermore, the time needed to reach the plateau level when digitoxin is given in maintenance dose form is one month as it is in normal patients. This implies that digitoxin half-life is not prolonged in uremic patients.[49] Indeed, digitoxin elimination may be considered normal in the face of renal failure.[50,51]

In patients with the nephrotic syndrome, digitoxin binding is decreased and there is a decrease in half-life of digitoxin secondary to an increased availability of drug for renal excretion. The decreased half-life and increased volume of distribution implies that greater drug doses may be needed in individual patients; however, the decrease in binding dictates that for any given drug level there is an increased amount of free drug present.[52]

Dialysis does not significantly decrease the total body stores of digoxin or digitoxin in that digoxin is sparingly distributed in the plasma space and digitoxin is highly protein bound.[51,53,54] Dialysis patients did not show impaired absorption of digitoxin but did show higher digoxin levels secondary to their renal failure.[51] It is suggested that digoxin be given at 0.125 mg/dl, 5 days per week and that digitoxin be given at 0.1 mg/dl 5 days per week to uremic patients undergoing dialysis. The serum half-lives of digoxin and digitoxin approximate each other in renal failure and 30 days are needed to reach a plateau concentration when these drugs are started in maintenance form or a change in drug dosage occurs. These dose levels will result in a low therapeutic, nontoxic serum concentration for digoxin of 0.84 ± 0.05 ng/ml and for digitoxin of 19 ± 1 ng/ml. No glycoside was given on the day of dialysis to avoid increasing body glycoside stores in the face of the electrolyte shifts that occur during dialysis. Heparin used with dialysis alters the binding of glycosides to serum proteins. Following renal transplantation digoxin clearance parallels the overall renal function of the patient.[55]

High performance liquid chromatography (HPLC) is able to detect trace quantities of digoxin metabolites in dialysis patients whereas patients with lesser degrees of renal impairment negligible quantities of digoxin metabolites were observed. In dialysis patients, if the RIA of digoxin with HPLC separation is related to the RIA of digoxin without prior separation, the ratio is less than 1. The ratio is greater than 1 when renal function is greater than 50 ml/min. Gibson concludes that the conventional RIA method for digoxin assay may overestimate digoxin concentrations in dialysis patients.[56]

One of the debates in literature concerning therapeutics has been whether digoxin or digitoxin is the preferred glycoside in renal failure. Obviously, digitoxin is less altered by renal failure, however, digoxin is altered in a reasonably predictable manner. If the clinical pharmacology of both agents is known in health and in renal failure, there is probably no clear cut preference if the usual clinical cautions are used.

ANTIARRHYTHMICS

Propranolol

Propranolol, a nonselective beta-adrenergic antagonist is used primarily in the adjunctive treatment of patients with hypertension, angina pectoris, and cardiac arrhythmias. When administered orally, propranolol undergoes a first-pass hepatic extraction and is metabolized by the hepatic oxidative pathway, specifically by hydroxylation to 4-hydroxy-propranolol. In subjects with normal renal function, propranolol is well absorbed when taken orally; due to the avid hepatic binding, oral doses result in lower plasma concentrations than equivalent intravenous doses. In addition, long term administration of propranolol results in hepatic saturation, which results in higher plasma concentrations and a prolongation of the biologic half-life.[57] There is significant inter-individual variability in the plasma concentration dose relationship, as well as significant intra-individual variability in plasma concentrations, depending upon the relationship between the administration of the dose and the mean consumed.[58,59] In addition, there is variability in the plasma propranolol concentration due to technical interference with vacutainer-type tubes[60] as well as with heparin.[61] This results in low plasma concentrations of propranolol and possibly erroneous interpretation of results.

Previous studies[62] in our laboratory have demonstrated no impairment to absorption in patients with chronic renal disease when compared with that in normal subjects and, of great interest, have demonstrated significantly higher plasma concentrations of propranolol within 1.5 hours after the administration of 80 mg. Following the administration of the same dosage to normal volunteer subjects, the peak plasma concentration was approximately one-third that obtained in patients, and it occurred at approximately 2.5 hours after the dose was given (Fig. 1). In the patient group, the dose per kilogram was significantly greater, yet the metabolic clearance was lower when compared with that in the control group. The fraction of the dose absorbed that is apparently available to the circulation and the fraction truly available to the circulation for pharmacologic effect were significantly greater in the patients with chronic renal insufficiency. Elimination half-life and the elimination rate constant (Table 3) were not significantly different in either group, yet because of the significantly higher plasma concentrations of propranolol, the area under the curve (AUC) was significantly greater by threefold (Table 4). It was concluded from these data that there was an impairment to the first-pass effect in the group with renal insufficiency. On the basis of our data, hepatic extraction and, therefore, clearance of propranolol are reduced in chronic renal disease.[62,63] These observations in addition to the greater dosage per unit weight (mg/kg), may explain the early, higher plasma levels and AUC observed in the patients with renal disease. Because of the first-pass phenomenon, less drug normally reaches the systemic circulation, and the calculation of the volume of distribution based on oral dosing would be theoretically inaccurate. A decrease in red blood cell mass, the decrease or absence of anatomic renal tissue, and loss of muscle mass (and, therefore, body weight) from

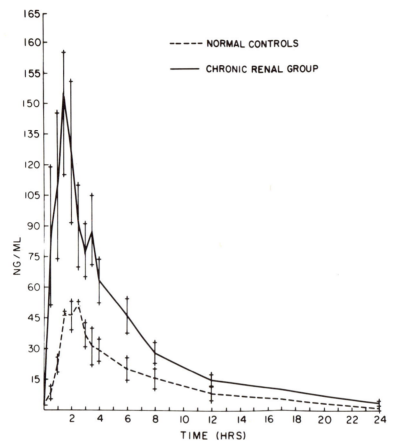

Figure 1. Propranolol concentrations in normal subjects (broken line) and in patients with end-stage renal failure (solid line) after the administration of a single dose of 80 ng.

chronic renal disease all contribute to a decrease in the volume of distribution in patients with end-stage renal disease. These facts, too, may explain the high AUC in the patient group. In fact, we have recently found a difference in the volume of distribution between patients with normal renal function and two patients with end-stage renal disease (Table 4) when given propranolol 1 mg/min IV for 10 minutes. The uremics have a contracted volume of distribution for propranolol.

When propranolol is given in long term maintenance doses (that is, 40 mg every 6 hours; 80 mg every 8 hours), the elimination half-life is shorter than when the drug is given in single doses[64] (Fig. 2, Table 3). There is evidence that certain drugs, for example, antipyrine,[65] diphenylhydan-

TABLE 3. Single dose pharmacokinetics of oral antiarrhythmics

	Propranolol*	Procainamide*	Quinidine*	Phenytoin†	Disopyramide*
			Normal Subjects		
T ½ (hr)	4.4	3.5	7.2	0.7	4.4
Elimination rate constant, Ke ($hr^{-1}B$)	0.157	0.198	0.096	0.05	0.16
			Patients with End-Stage Renal Disease		
T ½	3.2	12.8 (N)‡	6.6	1.4	8.3
Ke (B)	0.216	19.3 (A)§	0.105	0.1	0.08

* Active metabolite. See text.
† T ½ is shorter when drug is given in multiple doses.
‡ Physiologic anephric.
§ Anatomic anephric.

TABLE 4. Comparison of mean pharmacokinetic parameters: normal volunteers and patients with end-stage renal disease receiving propranolol, 80 mg

Dose/kg	Peak Concentration (ng/ml)	AUC (ng/ml × hr)	Metabolic clearance* (L/min)	fs†	F‡
Control Group					
1.05 ± 0.5	51.6 ± 1.0	274 ± 49	0.817 ± 0.039	0.254 ± 0.04	0.158 ± 0.02
Patients with End-Stage Renal Disease					
1.44 ± 0.2	155 ± 40	716 ± 149	0.637 ± 0.04	0.440 ± 0.05	0.275 ± 0.03
P <0.01	P <0.05	P <0.05	P <0.05	P <0.05	P <0.05

*Metabolic clearance $= \dfrac{FXD}{AVC}$

†$fs = \dfrac{Q}{Q + \dfrac{D-T}{AVC}}$ where Q = hepatic blood Flow of 1.1 L/min
T = 30 mg, threshold dose
D = 80 mg dose

‡$F = fs \dfrac{(D-T)}{D}$

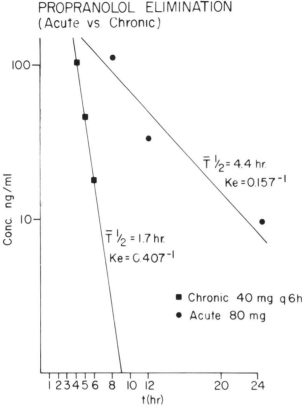

Figure 2. Propranolol elimination in patients with end-stage renal disease receiving long term therapy, 40 mg every 6 hr (solid box), versus those receiving a single dose of 80 mg (solid circles).

toin,[66] pentobarbital,[67] and other drugs that proceed through the oxidation process have unimpaired or even accelerated rates of elimination and normal to shortened biologic half-lives in patients with end-stage renal disease. It is likely that propranolol may be added to this list when the drug is given over a long period. These data may reflect an increase in the activity of the microsomal oxidation system in chronic renal failure. Steady-stage concentrations of propranolol in end-stage renal disease vary from patient to patient, dose to dose, and depend considerably on the relationship between the mean consumed and when blood is drawn for determining the concentration of the drug.

Based on this information, the initial dose of propranolol need not be reduced. Careful attention must be paid to blood pressure and pulse rate change as a result of the early elevated plasma concentrations. That the increased plasma propranolol is transient is demonstrated by a short $T\frac{1}{2}$ and when long term dosing is prescribed no accumulation of propranolol occurs. However, 4-hydroxypropranolol, naphthoxylactic acid, and naphthoxyacetic acid accumulation may occur but should not result in adverse or overt hemodynamic alterations.[68,69] Therefore, dosage alteration is unnecessary for chronic propranolol therapy in patients with ESRD.

Protein binding studies in our laboratory with radioactive carbon ^{14}C labelled propranolol or unlabelled drug, by means of ultracentrifugation and equilibrium dialysis, demonstrate that the binding of propranolol is not impaired in patients with renal insufficiency. However, when patients are treated with long term peritoneal dialysis, the binding of propranolol is significantly less; this is probably due to the loss of albumin during the peritoneal dialysis procedure. Because of its avid protein binding of 90 percent or greater, it can be predicted that the dialyzability of the drug is small. Previous work has demonstrated that this is the case with propranolol.[62]

Quinidine

Quinidine undergoes oxidation in the liver to several hydroxy derivatives. With normal renal function, renal excretion is rapid and 10 to 50 percent of a given quinidine dose is found unchanged in the urine within 24 hours of administration. The urinary excretion of quinidine is enhanced by acidification and delayed by alkalinization of the urine.[70] The half-life of quinidine has been shown to be the same in normal subjects, in patients with impaired renal function, and in those with congestive heart failure, a mean of 7 hours after a single dose of quinidine.[71] Previous studies[71] have contended that in patients with impaired renal function, the administration of doses equal to those given to normal persons resulted in higher plasma levels, but the nonspecificity of the assay techniques resulted in the measurement of quinidine and its polar metabolites. More recently, improved assay methodology has resulted in the measurement of the parent quinidine as well as the metabolites. Studies by Drayer and associates[73] have demonstrated in animal models the activity of 3-hydroxyquinidine, 2-oxoquinidinone, and the least active metabolite, O-desmethylquinidine. Quinidine, 3 (OH) and 2 (OXO) are equally potent antiarrhythmic drugs. In addition, both quinidine *and metabolites* may contribute to adverse effects if accumulation is detected in patients with ESRD.

Figure 3 shows plasma quinidine concentrations measured by double extraction method in steady-state studies. The concentrations of the drug are within the normal therapeutic range in patients with renal insuffi-

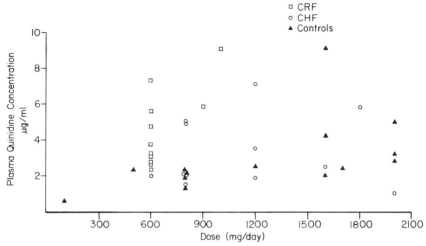

Figure 3. Plasma quinidine concentrations measured by the double-extraction method under steady state conditions. CRF = chronic renal failure; CHF = congestive heart failure.

ciency, in patients with congestive heart failure, and in control subjects being treated only for arrhythmia. The biologic half-life of quinidine following its long term use appears longer than that following a single dose.[73] This may be a reflection of rapid tissue uptake, avid tissue binding, and slow release following long term quinidine administration. At equilibrium, tissue to serum concentration ratios may be as large as 20.

Quinidine is 80 percent protein bound, and this binding is not altered in patients with impaired renal function. It is unlikely that the drug is dialyzable because of this phenomenon. However, since the therapeutic concentrations of quinidine in end-stage renal failure do not exceed the normal range, this antiarrhythmic may be safer to administer than procainamide. Dosage adjustments are advised during maintenance therapy because of the accumulation of metabolites. The initial dose may be unchanged but at a GFR less than 50 ml/min, maintenance dosage of 100 mg q4–8 hours, albeit restrictive, is therapeutic.

Procainamide

Procainamide is acetylated to n-acetylprocainamide (NAPA), an active metabolite. Contrary to previous data, urinary acidification does not increase the renal excretion of procainamide and, consequently, does not lower the half-life of the drug.[74] In patients with renal disease, urinary excretion of procainamide decreases proportionately with creatinine clearance. The biotransformation process of procainamide takes on great significance as the elimination of parent compound decreases (that is, as impairment of renal function progresses). Biotransformation becomes relatively more important when renal function is impaired due to the fact that the major metabolite, n-acetylprocainamide, is a potent active antiarrhythmic.[15,75]

There is no impairment to procainamide absorption in chronic renal insufficiency and the plasma concentration peak within 1.5 to 2 hours after a single dose of 500 mg.[76] The normal half-life of the drug is 3.5 to 4 hours, and this can be prolonged three to fourfold in patients with impaired renal function (Table 3). Normally, the drug is only 15 percent protein bound and is readily dialyzable. With long term administration, there is a prolonged half-life which is within the same range as that following a single dose (9 to 19 hours), but the biologic half-life of the n-acetylprocainamide metabolite is so long as to be indeterminate.[15] N-acetylprocainamide is present in significant concentrations in the plasma of patients taking procainamide for more than one to two days.[15] It has an antiarrhythmic activity similar to procainamide in animal models and in man.[77,78] Over 85 percent of a dose of n-acetylprocainamide in man is excreted unchanged in the urine.

Measurement of plasma concentrations of procainamide by the usual fluorometic or colorimetric methods does not detect the pharmacologically active n-acetylprocainamide. In patients with high n-acetylprocainamide levels (patients in whom drugs acetylate rapidly or patients with renal failure who are receiving long term procainamide therapy), determination of procainamide levels alone by these methods can cause misleading blood level interpretations. The acetylator phenotype can be determined by using the n-acetylprocainamide concentration ratio in plasma. Assuming that the procainamide has been given for three or more days and that the plasma is obtained 3 hours after the administration of a dose of procainamide, the ratio is below 0.85 in slow acetylators and above 1.0 in rapid acetylators. A slow acetylator would have high concentration of procainamide and low concentrations of n-acetylprocainamide, and the reverse would obtain in patients who are rapid acetylators. In patients with renal failure, studied on nondialysis days, the lack of decline in n-acetylprocainamide plasma levels might be due to 1) n-acetylprocainamide being synthesized from the procainamide still present and 2) impaired renal excretion of n-acetylprocainamide in these patients, since n-acetylprocainamide is eliminated mainly by renal excretion. Since the n-acetylprocainamide accumulates in patients with poor renal function, both n-acetylprocainamide and procainamide concentrations should be monitored in these patients.[15] The maintenance dosage of procainamide probably should be lowered and the dosing interval extended (instead of q8 hours, dose at q12 hours), commensurate with maintenance of good arrhythmia control, as the n-acetylprocainamide accumulates. In patients with renal failure, the acetylator phenotype cannot be determined on the basis of measuring n-acetylprocainamide and procainamide plasma ratios as is done for nonazotemic cardiac patients because of this accumulation.

In our present state of knowledge, with regard to the safety of antiarrhythmics in patients with chronic renal failure, it appears that quinidine is the drug of choice for treatment of patients with atrial and ventricular arrhythmias.

Lidocaine

The use of lidocaine in chronic renal insufficiency is not unique and is confined primarily to patients with cardiovascular complications. It is used often as a local anesthetic for minor surgical procedures as well as in treating uremic pruritis,[79] and in customary doses has not created or been associated with any adverse reactions. Lidocaine is metabolized by the liver via an oxidative pathway through N-dealkylation to monoethylglycinexylidide (MEGX) and glycinexylidide (GX), which are active metabolites.[80] It has a biphasic elimination process, and a short and a long half-life: in subjects with chronic renal insufficiency 9.3 min and 77 min respectively as compared with 8.3 min and 108 min in normal control subjects.[81] MEGX and GX are active metabolites (local anesthetic, antiarrhythmic, hypotensive, and central nervous system toxic properties), but only GX can accumulate in patients with chronic renal insufficiency and create adverse pharmacologic responses.[134] Normally, lidocaine is 60 percent bound and this is concentration dependent. Its binding and dialyzability in patients with renal insufficiency have not been studied. The areas of systemic disease in which patients with end-stage renal disease might be subject to adverse reactions from both lidocaine and its metabolites are in acute myocardial infarction with arrhythmias, congestive heart failure with right sided complications, and in chronic or acute hepatic insufficiency.[81,82] Because the drug is normally metabolized by the liver and undergoes a first-pass effect similar to that of propranolol, 65 percent of the drug is extracted on the first pass, leaving 35 percent free (of which 40 percent is unbound to protein) to act pharmacologically in the system.[83,84] If this first-pass extraction by the liver is deranged because of primary or secondary hepatic involvement, metabolic processes involving lidocaine might be slowed and cumulative effects of the drug might be profound. If chronic renal disease results in an impairment to the first-pass effect, an increase in the parent drug and possibly free drug concentration may become apparent and, therefore, account for accelerated metabolism and a shorter half-life. However, there is rationale for dosage reduction in patients with ESRD in order to avoid toxicity due to retention of GX.

Disopyramide (Norpace)[85]

Oral administration of disopyramide as the phosphate salt or free base results in rapid and nearly complete absorption. The relative systemic availability of the two oral forms has varied between studies but appears to be approximately 70 to 85 percent compared with intravenous administration. Disopyramide undergoes limited hepatic first-pass metabolism, that is, approximately 16 percent. The extent of protein binding of disopyramide shows wide interpatient variability and is concentration dependent. The fraction not bound to plasma proteins increases with total plasma concentration and plasma clearance is independent of the concentration of the free drug. This results in the concentration of free or unbound drug increasing proportionally with dose, but total drug concentration shows a less than proportionate increase.

Peak plasma concentrations which were lower in patients with acute myocardial infarction, that is, less than 1 μg/ml than in healthy subjects (2 to 3 μg/ml) receiving the same dose occurred approximately 2 hr after oral administration of 100 mg. The intravenous administration of 1.5 to 2 mg/kg results in a rapid peak in disopyramide plasma concentrations, declining immediately after injection to about 4 μg/ml at 5 min, the distribution half-life being approximately 3 min in healthy subjects but 5 times prolonged in patients with recent myocardial infarction. The steady-state volume of distribution after intravenous administration was greater in healthy subjects (40 to 89 L) than in patients with acute myocardial infarction (33 to 60 L) but appear to be slightly reduced in patients with impaired renal function.

Approximately 50 to 60 percent of an administered dose is excreted unchanged with the majority being eliminated in the urine and a small amount in the feces. Disopyramide undergoes N-dealkylation as the primary metabolic pathway and the major metabolite is excreted by the kidney. In animals the N-dealkylated metabolite has some antiarrhythmic activity but was less active than disopyramide. The elimination half-life after intravenous administration was longer in patients with recent myocardial infarction (7 to 11.8 hr) or severe renal dysfunction (8.3 to 43 hr, the value increasing as renal function worsens) and shortest in healthy subjects (4.4 to 8.2 hr). Similarily, an oral dose of 200 to 300 mg was excreted more slowly in patients with ventricular arrhythmias (half-life of 9.3 to 33.8 hr) than in healthy volunteers (8.2 to 8.9 hr).

Previous studies of disopyramide kinetics in normal subjects have shown a total clearance can vary from 60 to 200 ml/min.[86] It has been demonstrated that disopyramide clearance only falls significantly when the creatinine clearance has dropped to 20 to 25 ml/min. The half-life then becomes prolonged and may be 5 times that found with normal renal function. Dosage modification is then essential to avoid excessive plasma concentrations.[87]

Therefore, it appears prudent to alter the dosage of disopyramide in patients with impaired renal function and to reinforce this reduction in dosage and/or prolong the dosage interval when the combined disease entities of acute myocardial infarction and chronic renal failure coincide. Studies correlating plasma levels of disopyramide with clinical effects are limited but it appears that a plasma concentration of approximately 3 to 6 μg/ml represents a desirable therapeutic range.

If one assumes an average plasma concentration of 4 μg/ml with patients with normal renal function showing a half-life of 7 to 8 hours, the disopyramide dose should be 150 to 200 mg every 6 hours. Whitting and Elliott[85] have suggested that in patients whose creatinine clearance is less than 8 ml/min, the dose would be 150 mg every 24 hours or 75 mg every 12 hr or 50 mg every 8 hr. For patients with less severe renal impairment, the dosage might be 150 mg every 12 hours or 100 mg every 8 hours.[87] Disopyramide dialyzability has been demonstrated in vitro using human blood containing an initial plasma concentration of 22 mg/L which was then dialyzed at body temperature in a Cordis-Dow number 4 artificial kidney at a blood flow rate of 250 ml/min and the disopyramide plasma concentration fell to 3 mg/L within 2 hours. Karim[88] concluded that, based on the in vitro data, hemodialysis may be of potential use in enhancing the elimination of toxic concentrations of disopyramide from the body.

Disopyramide has anticholinergic activity which may result in dryness of the mouth and difficulty in urination. Patients with impaired renal function receiving disopyramide may alter their fluid intake as a consequence of dryness of the mouth and those that are still able to produce urine may have difficulty in doing so if there is urinary retention. Rarely, peripheral neuropathy as well as pruritus may develop in patients receiving disopyramide and this may complicate existing peripheral neuropathy.

Phenytoin (Dilantin)[8-13]

Phenytoin absorption in renal failure is normal and plasma concentrations are adequate for anticonvulsant and antiarrhythmic activity even when reduced dosages of the drug are administered. Phenytoin kinetics are dose dependent in that the more that is given the more hepatic saturation occurs and the more prolonged the half-life that is observed. However, these kinetics are substantially different in patients with impaired renal function. It was observed that plasma concentrations as low as 2 μg/ml, which ordinarily is subtherapeutic (10 to 20 μg/ml is normal therapeutic range), were effective in reducing seizure activity after routine dosage was given to patients with impaired renal function. This in fact was also sufficient to produce symptoms of phenytoin toxicity namely nystagmus and ataxia. Reidenberg and colleagues[66] have demonstrated that with advancing renal impairment total plasma concentration of phenytoin decreases owing to greater degrees of unbinding of phenytoin. That is, as renal function deteriorates the plasma protein binding of phenytoin decreases resulting in more free drug not only for pharmacologic activity but to be metabolized by the liver. It has also been demonstrated that in normal subjects phenytoin is extensively metabolized to a hydroxy metabolite which is conjugated to glucuronide and excreted by the kidney. This has little if any pharmacologic activity as an anticonvulsant or a sedative. It has been shown to accumulate, however, in patients with renal insufficiency. In patients with impaired renal function, the plasma half-life of phenytoin is shortened most likely because there is more free drug to be metabolized by the liver.

Patients with impaired renal function have abnormalities in carbohydrate metabolism regardless of whether or not they are diabetic. Phenytoin has been demonstrated to impair insulin release.[89] Phenytoin, likewise, interacts with vitamin D, and this may result in hypocalcemia, hypophosphatemia, and clinical manifestation of rickets.[89,90] The latter metabolic problem may compromise the existing renal osteodystrophy and secondary hyperparathyroidism. When given with digitoxin, phenytoin can induce the metabolism of this glycoside. This results in more digoxin being produced and a shortening of the digitoxin half-life. The increase in free phenytoin in uremia can certainly explain such an interaction.[91] Serum quinidine levels are reduced and its half-life shortened by phenytoin and phenobarbital.[92] There appears to be no need to alter the dosage of phenytoin in patients with renal impairment, although the therapeutic and toxic effects may be seen at lower plasma concentrations owing to the protein binding abnormalities.

The dialyzability of phenytoin is insignificant. This is probably related to the fact that of the total amount of phenytoin ingested, small amounts (less than 10 percent) of unchanged phenytoin are excreted in the urine and feces, while 60 to 80 percent is excreted in the urine as the parahydroxy derivative or glucuronide conjugate.[93,94]

ANTIHYPERTENSIVES

The treatment of hypertension in end-stage renal disease will be covered in a subsequent chapter. The purpose of this section is to summarize the pharmacokinetic and dosage data of the antihypertensives given to patients with renal insufficiency.

Thiazide Diuretics[95,96]

All thiazides are readily absorbed in the gastrointestinal tract (25 to 50 percent) and have a diuretic effect within 1 hour following administration. All diuretics including the long acting metolazone and chlorthalidone are handled by renal elimination (excretion) with negligible hepatic biotransformation. However, the thiazides lose their efficacy as diuretics when the creatinine clearance is less than 30 ml/min. Chlorothiazide is 60 percent bound to plasma albumin. Since these agents are not used when the glomerular filtration rate is less than 30 ml/min, the exact knowledge concerning dosage restriction in advanced renal failure and the dialysance are not available. Metolazone added to furosemide may produce some added effect.

Furosemide

Furosemide is the diuretic of choice in complicated hypertension when associated with edema and/or azotemia. It has a prolonged half-life in patients with impaired renal function and its elimination is mainly by renal mechanisms. The plasma protein binding of this organic acid is impaired in end-stage renal disease and thus more free furosemide is available for pharmacologic activity. Its dialyzability is poor.[97,98]

Mitchell[99] has elegantly demonstrated that furosemide can be transformed in the liver to toxic metabolites which when combined covalently with tissue macromolecules cause significant necrosis in the lungs, liver, and kidneys of experimental animals. Clinically, there have been no cases reported of pulmonary or hepatic damage but there is evidence of interstitial nephritis secondary to furosemide and, in these particular instances, the patients were azotemic.[100]

Because of the prolonged biological half-life and potentially prolonged duration of action in renal failure, it is wise to restrict the dosage to a maximum of between 200 to 400 mg/day and if this does not produce the desired effect then in the instance where renal function is so severely impaired, dialysis would be the wise alternative to avoid adverse reactions.

Propranolol

This has been covered in the section on antiarrhythmics

OTHER BETA-ADRENOCEPTOR BLOCKING AGENTS

Timolol

Timolol[101] is 6 times as potent as propranolol with no cardiac selectivity or membrane stabilizing activity. Timolol is only 10 percent protein bound. Its elimination kinetics are superimposable regardless of renal function with an elimination half-life in patients with renal disease approximating 4 hr and this compares with similar half-life in patients with normal renal function.[101] Following 20 mg of timolol given in single dose, there does seem to be a prolongation of the blood pressure response as well as heart rate response with the systolic and diastolic pressure and heart rate very gradually returning to predosing levels by 24 hours. When given prior to hemodialysis, there are significant hemodynamic effects leading to hypotension, bradycardia, nausea, and sweating. These effects would contraindict the use of timolol prior to dialysis.[101] Timolol does not give rise to active metabolites in contrast to propranolol which does give rise to an active metabolite.

Labetalol

Labetalol is an investigational antihypertensive agent with both alpha and beta adrenoreceptor blocking properties. It is extensively metabolized in the liver with less than 5 percent being excreted unchanged in the urine. Based on this fact it would be safe to give the patient with chronic renal disease. However, bioavailability studies with labetalol demonstrated that there was increased bioavailability in patients with chronic liver disease owing to a reduction in first pass metabolism.[102,103] This correlated negatively with serum albumin concentrations. In addition, the decrease in heart rate and blood pressure was greater after oral administration suggesting an exaggerated response due to the increased bioavailability. Similar results have been reported with increased bioavailability for propranolol. Oxyprenolol, alprenolol, and metoprolol which also have high hepatic extraction have not yet been studied in this setting of chronic hepatic disease but similar results might be anticipated.

Pindolol

Pindolol is 6 times as potent as propranolol and its major advantage is that is has significant partial agonist activity. Its half-life in normal renal function is 3 to 4 hours and 40 percent of a single dose of pindolol is recovered unchanged in the urine.[104,105] Despite this, there has not been any correlation found between the overall elimination rate constant of pindolol and endogenous creatinine clearance. Ohnhaus and associates[104] concluded that the extrarenal elimination rate constant was increased. However, Øie and Levy[105] found a statistically significant positive correlation between the renal clearance of pindolol and creatinine.

Sotalol[106]

Sotalol which is approximately one-tenth to one-third as potent as propranolol and has no cardioselectivity, partial agonist activity, or membrane stabilizing activity, is excreted mainly by the kidneys as unchanged drug, and in patients with end-stage renal disease the plasma half-life is approximately 42 hr as compared with 5 hr in normal subjects. Thus, significant dosage reduction and widening of dosage interval is suggested.

Metoprolol

Metoprolol is 12 percent protein bound and has primarily hepatic biotransformation with some first-pass effect. The half-life of oral metoprolol in normal subjects is 3 to 4 hr and about 3 percent of a dose is recovered unchanged in the urine. There are no active metabolites, and to date, although pharmacokinetics have not been performed in impaired renal function, there seems to be no need to alter the dosage in patients with impaired renal function.[107] Interestingly, about 95 percent of an oral or intravenous dose of metoprolol is recovered in the urine over a period of 72 hours. The elimination half-life of the total metabolites after oral administration is about 3 hr, but after an intravenous dose is about 5 hr, indicating that the route of administration might influence the metabolic pathways of metoprolol. This phenomenon might reflect the first-pass elimination which metoprolol is subjected to resulting in 50 percent of administered dose reaching the systemic circulation.

Alprenolol[108]

When compared to propranolol, alprenolol has less bioavailability (10 percent) and is avidly protein bound with a similar elimination half-life as propranolol. Less than 1 percent of the drug is excreted unchanged, and like propranolol it too has active metabolites. It is nonselective and equipotent to propranolol but it does have greater partial agonist activity. Although pharmacokinetics of alprenolol have not been delineated in patients with impaired renal function, the fact that hepatic biotransformation gives rise to an active metabolite would suggest that a dosage reduction should be recommended in order to avoid significant accumulation of the active metabolite. This recommendation would apply in advanced renal failure and careful observation of pharmacodynamic activity would be necessary.

Atenolol[108]

Atenolol has an elimination half-life in subjects with normal renal function of 6 to 9 hours. It is equipotent to propranolol, it is cardio-selective, and only a small amount crosses the blood brain barrier. There are no active metabolites and approximately 40 percent of atenolol is recovered unchanged in the urine following a single dose. Multiple dose studies suggest that dosage reduction should be employed if given to patients with impaired renal function, that is, no change in dose for a creatinine clearance range of 125 to 35 ml/min. At 35 to 15 ml/min, instead of the usual 100 mg/day, give 50 mg/day or 100 mg every 2 days. For creative clearances under 15 ml/min, give a 25 mg daily dose or any dosage interval lengthened to 100 mg every 4 days or 50 mg every 2 days.

Nadolol[109,110]

Nadolol is a noncardioselective beta adrenergic blocking agent which has the longest plasma half-life of any known beta blocking drug and thus can be administered once daily. It is 2 to 4 times as potent as propranolol; it is only about 30 percent protein bound; more than 90 percent is recovered in the urine and feces unchanged; as a result there are no active metabolites. Its half-life in patients with normal renal function is 17 to 24 hours following a single oral dose. The renal clearance of nadolol has been found to correlate with creatinine clearance; and, as a consequence, the plasma half-life is prolonged in patients with impaired renal function. Therefore, dosage intervals in patients with decreased renal function receiving nadolol should have the dosage adjusted according to the creatinine clearance. Hemodialysis can effectively reduce serum concentrations of the drug and thus be useful as a means of treating nadolol intoxication. The best way to achieve dosage reduction is that when creatinine clearance is below 50 ml/min the dosage can be reduced in half and the dosage interval can be widened to every other day.

ANGIOTENSIN II ANTAGONIST (SARALASIN) AND CONVERTING ENZYME INHIBITOR (CAPTOPRIL)

The elimination half-life of saralasin in hypertensive man is 3.2 min.[111] The pharmacologic half-life as determined by the rate of return of blood pressure after saralasin induced reduction in blood pressure is approximately 8 min.[111] There was a brief time required to reach steady state plasma concentrations with saralasin and a plateau is achieved in a 15 min period.[111] There is no data to date on the elimination kinetics of saralasin in patients with impaired renal function. In view of its brief duration of action in subjects with normal renal function, the angiotensin II antagonist probably does not accumulate to any significant degree in impaired renal function. The effect of saralasin on blood pressure and on hemodynamics in patients with terminal renal failure has been studied. The fall in blood pressure in patients demonstrated that high renin and angiotensin levels may be involved in the pathogenesis of hypertension in some patients with terminal renal failure.[112] Although pharmacokinetic data are incomplete for captopril, its clinical effect has been studied in the hypertension of chronic renal failure. In those patients studied the drug was well tolerated without any adverse effect in the majority or dosage restriction necessary. Patients with impaired renal function have tolerated maintenance doses of 200 mg, 2 times a day, but in some proteinuria, skin rash, loss of taste (aqeusia) and agranulocytosis have been reported.[113,136] When nonmalignant or accelerated hypertension exists, prior dialysis or furosemide dosing will effect a more potent antihypertensive response to saralasin or captopril.

METHYLDOPA

Methyldopa is metabolized in the liver to two active metabolites, alphamethyldopamine and alphamethylnorepinephrine. These metabolites can accumulate in the azotemic patient and may account for some exaggeration of the drowsiness and somnolence which methyldopa can cause in patients with normal renal function. The half-life is increased in renal failure but not to a prolonged duration, that is, from approximately 1.5 to a maximum 4 to 5 hours following a dosage of methyldopa.[114-116] Dosage alterations must be made on an individual basis depending on the patient's response.

The drug is dialyzable owing to the fact that it is minimally protein bound.[117] Dosage modification in the azotemic patient probably is not necessary until the creatinine clearance is less than 50 ml/min but must be individualized depending on the degree of side effects that can be observed. It is probably easier to widen the dosage interval from 6 to 12 hours than to decrease the drug dosage. It must also be pointed out that because Coombs' positive antibody to the red blood cell occurs in 20 to 35 percent of patients that the azotemic who is already anemic and may require transfusions may present a blood typing problem.

CLONIDINE[118,119,135]

Hepatic biotransformation accounts for approximately 50 percent of the elimination of clonidine; 50 percent of clonidine and its metabolites are excreted mainly through the kidneys. Peak plasma levels correlate positively with xerostomia and drowsiness. The antihypertensive effect may last beyond the half-life. The pharmacokinetics of clonidine in renal failure reveal that the elimination rate varies directly with the creatinine clearance. Prolongation of the elimination half-life of twice normal may be seen but clinically there appears to be no adverse effects with clonidine when given in customary doses to patients with renal insufficiency.[120] In nonazotemic serum the plasma protein binding of clonidine is 20 to 40 percent.[121] This suggests that the drug may be dialyzable. Yet studies using ^{14}C-clonidine do not confirm this contention. Dialysance of ^{14}C-clonidine removes approximately 5 percent of the total body stores. Thus, no significant dosage adjustments are required postdialysis.[121] There is a narrow therapeutic range (0.8 to 2.0 ng/ml) of plasma clonidine which beyond the upper limit *may* lead to peripheral alpha-constriction and a loss of control of blood pressure. This coincides with clonidine doses greater than 2 mg per day but *may* be seen in azotemics when higher concentrations are seen. The dryness of the mouth which may occur with clonidine and methyldopa may lead to an increase in fluid consumption affecting fluid balance in patients with ESRD.

PRAZOSIN

Prazosin is biotransformed in the liver to inactive metabolites. Its elimination kinetics are unaltered in renal insufficiency, produce no change in protein binding, slightly lower plasma concentrations and has an equivalent half-life in those with normal renal function.[122] When relating the effectiveness of prazosin in patients with normal and abnormal renal function at doses greater than 9 to 20 mg/day,[123] the drug does not seem to be as effective with diuretic alone and may need an additional boost from beta blockade or clonidine.

MINOXIDIL[124,137]

Minoxidil is biotransformed in the liver to inactive metabolites. Its elimination half-life is unaltered in patients with renal failure. The elimination half-life is the same whether the drug is given in single dosage or multiple dosage. The protein binding has not been studied nor has the dialyzability of minoxidil. Because the drug is extensively metabolized and does not depend on the kidney for its elimination, its dialyzability would be of no significance. There are no known adverse interactions between minoxidil and diuretics or bradycardic agents with which it must be coadministered. No dosage alterations are necessary in ESRD.

HYDRALAZINE

Hydralazine is biotransformed by hydroxylation, conjugation, and acetylation (in liver and small intestine). Only a small fraction is excreted unchanged in the urine. Yet hydralazine half-life is prolonged and plasma concentrations are higher in patients with renal failure.[125,126] Present evidence points to impaired (slowed) hepatic biotransformation as a cause for the higher plasma concentrations.[125] There is a greater prolongation of the half-life in those patients whose acetylation phenotype is slow.[126] There is no data which demonstrates any increase in the incidence of the lupus syndrome in slow acetylators with renal failure. Dosages of hydralazine must be individualized based on the therapeutic response (given with diuretic and bradycardic drugs).

DIAZOXIDE

Diazoxide is a potent direct acting vasodilator with an onset of action within minutes following a bolus injection.[127] Approximately 50 percent is excreted unchanged by the kidney.[128] In renal failure, the protein binding is diminished and its biologic half-life is prolonged.[129] There is poor correlation between the plasma levels of diazoxide and therapeutic response. The hypotensive effect is only one-third as long as its half-life (20 to 36 hours in normal subjects; prolonged in renal failure).[128] Diazoxide is dialyzable by hemo and peritoneal dialysis.

NITROPRUSSIDE[130]

Nitroprusside is excreted fully metabolized in the urine. Thiocyanate is an end-product of nitroprusside metabolism. Normally, the half-life of nitroprusside is 3 to 4 min. This is prolonged in azotemia. In renal failure adequate diuresis or dialysis must be maintained in order to prevent toxic accumulation of the centrally depressing metabolite, thiocyanate.

GUANETHIDINE

Guanethidine may be prescribed without dosage alteration in uremic patients.[131,132] The metabolites may accumulate if not excreted, but their activity is negligible. *However,* because it produces severe orthostatic hypotension, impotence, significant reductions in cardiac output and renal blood flow, and inhibits compensatory circulatory reflexes during ultrafiltration with dialysis, it must be used with extreme caution.

RESERPINE

Owing to its central depressing activity, reserpine should seldom be used in patients with or without renal failure. It is extensively metabolized in the liver and only when renal function is at 10 percent of normal is there any cumulation of reserpine.

Finally, the areas of biotransformation and pharmacokinetics involve at times drug-drug interactions. These interactions may be pharmacodynamic (propranolol-isoproterenol) or pharmacokinetic (warfarin-phenobarbital). At present, there is no information (other than anecdotal) concerning interactions unique to renal failure that is not documented for the patient with normal renal function. As noted above, alterations in biotransformation, including plasma protein binding, in renal disease may lead to untoward reactions in patients receiving multiple drug regimens. Physician awareness of the changes in the principles of drug biotransformation in disease states may prevent interactions from becoming clinically significant. Additional supplemental information can be found in Table 1.

In conjunction with drug therapy, dialytic treatment may be necessary to supplement the effects of these pharmacologic agents or in fact to remove toxic levels of these drugs. The principles of dialysis in patients with heart disease are addressed in Chapter 4.

REFERENCES

1. Smith, J.W., Seidl, L.G., and Cluff, L.E.: Studies on the epidemiology of adverse drug reactions, V. Clinical factors influencing susceptibility. Ann. Intern. Med. 65:629, 1966.
2. Reidenberg, M.M.: Renal Function and Drug Action. W.B. Saunders, Philadelphia, 1971.
3. Lindner, A., Charra, B., Sherrard, D.J., et al.: Accelerated atherosclerosis in prolonged maintenance hemodialysis. N. Engl. J. Med. 290:697, 1974.

4. Bennet, W.M., Muther, R.S. and Parker, R.A.: Drug therapy in renal failure: dosing guidelines in four adults. Part 2. Ann. Intern. Med. 93:286, 1980.

5. Lowenthal, D.T., Affrime, M.B., and Piraino, A.J.: Drug distribution in renal failure. Drug Metabol. Rev. In Press.

6. Gibaldi, M.: Drug distribution in renal failure. Am. J. Med. 62:471, 1977.

7. Reidenberg, M.M.: The binding of drugs to plasma proteins and the interpretation of measurements of plasma concentrations of drugs in patients with poor renal function. Am. J. Med. 62:466, 1977.

8. Reidenberg, M.M., and Affrime, M.B.: Influence of disease on binding of drugs to plasma proteins. Ann. N.Y. Acad. Sci. 226:115, 1973.

9. Reidenberg, M.M.: The biotransformation of drugs in renal failure. Am. J. Med. 62:482, 1977.

10. Letteri, J.M., Mellk, H., Louis, S., et al.: Diphenylhydantoin metabolism in uremia. N. Engl. J. Med. 285:648, 1970.

11. Odar-Cederlof, I., and Borga, O.: Kinetics of diphenylhydantoin in uraemic patients: consequences of decreased protein binding. Europ. J. Clin. Pharmacol. 7:31, 1974.

12. Odar-Cederlof, I.: Studies on the plasma protein binding of drugs in patients with renal failure. Thesis, Karolinska Institutet, Stockholm, Sweden, 1975.

13. Reynolds, F., Ziroyanis, P.N., Jones, N.F., et al.: Salivary phenytoin concentrations in epilepsy and in chronic renal failure. Lancet 2:384, 1976.

14. Szeto, H.H., Inturrisi, C.E., Houde, R., et al.: The accumulation of normeperidine, an active metabolite of meperidine, in patients with renal failure or cancer. Ann. Intern. Med. 86:738, 1977.

15. Drayer, D.E., Lowenthal, D.T., Woosley, R.L., et al.: Cumulation of N-acetylprocainamide, an active metabolite of procainamide, in patients with impaired renal function. Clin. Pharmacol. Ther. 22:63, 1977.

16. Drayer, D.E.: Active drug metabolites and renal failure. Am. J. Med. 62:486, 1977.

17. Reidenberg, M.M., and Drayer, D.E.: Drug metabolism and active drug metabolites in renal failure. J. Dialysis 1:313, 1977.

18. Dettli, L.: Individualization of drug dosage in patients with renal disease. Med. Clin. N. Am. 58:977, 1974.

19. Bennett, W.M., Singer, L., and Coggins, C.J.: A guide to drug therapy in renal failure. JAMA 230:1544, 1974.

20. Anderson, R.J., Gambertoglio, J.G., and Schrier, R.W.: Clinical Use of Drugs in Renal Failure. Charles C Thomas, Springfield, Ill., 1976.

21. Cheigh, J.S.: Drug administration in renal failure. Am. J. Med. 62:555, 1977.

22. Butler, T.C.: Termination of drug action by elimination of unchanged drug. Fed. Proc. 17:1158, 1958.

23. Beller, G.A., Smith, T.W., Abelmann, W.H., et al.: Digitalis intoxication. A prospective clinical study with serum level correlations. N. Engl. J. Med. 284:989, 1971.

24. Lasagna, L.: How useful are serum digitalis measurements? N. Engl. J. Med. 294:898, 1976.

25. Koch-Weser, J., Duhme, D.W., and Greenblatt, D.J.: Influence of serum digoxin concentration measurements on frequency of digitoxicity. Clin. Pharmacol. Ther. 16:284, 1973.

26. Duhme, D.W., Greenblatt, D.J., and Koch-Weser, J.: Reduction of digoxin toxicity associated with measurement of serum levels. Ann. Intern. Med. 80:516, 1974.

27. Jelliffe, R.W., Buell, J., and Kalaba, R.: Reduction of digitalis toxicity by

computer-assisted glycoside dosage regimens. Ann. Intern. Med. 77:891, 1972.

28. Doherty, J.E., Flanigan, W.J., Perkins, W.H., et al.: Studies with tritiated digoxin in anephric human subjects. Circulation 35:298, 1967.

29. Maloney, C., Ahmed, M., Tweeddale, M., et al.: Biotransformation and elimination of digoxin with normal and minimal renal function. Clin. Res. 24:651A, 1976.

30. Doherty, J.E., and Kane, J.J.: Clinical pharmacology of digitalis glycosides. Ann. Rev. Med. 26:159, 1975.

31. Doherty, J.E., Perkins, W.H., and Wilson, M.C.: Studies with tritiated digoxin in renal failure. Am. J. Med. 37:536, 1964.

32. Marcus, F.I., Peterson, A., Salel, A., et al.: The metabolism of tritiated digoxin in renal insufficiency in dogs and man. J. Pharm. Exp. Ther. 152:372, 1966.

33. Doherty, J.E., Bissett, J.K., Kane, J.J., et al.: Tritiated digoxin: studies in renal disease in human subjects. Int. J. Clin. Pharmacol. 12:89, 1975.

34. Gault, M.H., Jeffrey, J.R., Chirito, E., et al.: Studies of digoxin dosage, kinetics and serum concentrations in renal failure and review of the literature. Nephron 17:161, 1976.

35. Doherty, J.E., Flanigan, W.J., Patterson, R.M., et al.: The excretion of tritiated digoxin in normal human volunteers before and after unilateral nephrectomy. Circulation 40:555, 1969.

36. Blood, P.M., Nelp, W.B., Truell, S.H.: Relationship of the excretion of tritiated digoxin to renal function. Am. J. Med. Sci. 251:133, 1966.

37. Paulson, M.F., and Welling, P.G.: Calculation of serum digoxin levels in patients with normal and impaired renal function. J. Clin. Pharm. 16:660, 1976.

38. Marcus, F.I.: Current concepts of digoxin therapy. Mod. Concepts Cardiovasc. Dis. 45:77, 1976.

39. Reuning, R.H., Sams, R.A., and Notari, R.E.: Role of pharmacokinetics in drug dosage adjustment. 1. Pharmacologic effect kinetics and apparent volume of distribution of digoxin. J. Clin. Pharm. 13:127, 1973.

40. Jusko, W.J., Szefler, S.J., and Goldfarb, A.L.: Pharmacokinetic design of digoxin dosage regimens in relation to renal function. J. Clin. Pharm. 14:525, 1974.

41. Wagner, J.G., Yates, J.D., Willis, P.W., et al.: Correlation of plasma levels of digoxin in cardiac patients with dose and measures of renal function. Clin. Pharmacol. Ther. 15:291, 1974.

42. Halkin, H., Sheiner, L.B., and Melmon, K.L.: Determinants of the renal clearance of digoxin. Clin. Pharmacol. Ther. 17:385, 1975.

43. Koup, J.R., Jusko, W.J., Elwood, C.M., et al.: Digoxin pharmacokinetics: Role of renal failure in dosage regimen design. Clin. Pharmacol. Ther. 18:9, 1975.

44. Jelliffe, R.W.: A mathematical analysis of digitalis kinetics in patients with normal and reduced renal function. Math. Biosci. 1:305, 1965.

45. Jelliffe, R.W.: An improved method of digoxin therapy. Ann. Int. Med. 69:703, 1968.

46. Storstein, L.: Studies on digitalis. V. The influence of impaired renal function, hemodialysis and drug interaction on serum protein binding of digitoxin and digoxin. Clin. Pharmacol. Ther. 20:6, 1976.

47. Jelliffe, R.W., Buell, J., Kalaba, R., et al.: An improved method of digitoxin therapy. Ann. Intern. Med. 72:453, 1970.

48. Sheiner, L.B.: The use of serum concentrations of digitalis for quantitative therapeutic decisions. Cardiovasc. Clin. 6:141, 1974.

49. Rasmussen, K., Jervell, J., Storstein, L., et al.: Digitoxin kinetics in patients with impaired renal function. Clin. Pharmacol. Ther. 13:6, 1972.

50. Vohringer, H.F., Reitbrock, N., and Spurny, P.: Disposition of digitoxin in renal failure. Clin. Pharmacol. Ther. 19:387, 1976.

51. Finkelstein, F.O., Goffinet, J.A., Hendler, E.O., et al.: Pharmacokinetics of digoxin and digitoxin in patients undergoing hemodialysis. Am. J. Med. 58:525, 1975.

52. Storstein, L.: Studies on digitalis. VII. Influence of nephrotic syndrome on protein binding, pharmacokinetics, and renal excretion of digitoxin and cardioactive metabolites. Clin. Pharmacol. Ther. 20:158, 1976.

53. Ackerman, G.L., Doherty, J.E., and Flanigan, W.J.: Peritoneal dialysis and hemodialysis of tritiated digoxin. Ann. Intern. Med. 67:718, 1967.

54. Lukas, D.S., and DeMartino, A.G.: Binding of digoxin and some related cardenolides to human plasma proteins. J. Clin. Invest. 48:1041, 1969.

55. Doherty, J.E., Flanigan, W.J., and Perkins, W.H.: Tritiated digoxin excretion of patients following renal transplantation. Circulation 37:865, 1968.

56. Gibson, T.P., and Nelson, H.A.: Evidence for accumulation of digoxin metabolites in renal failure. Clin. Pharmacol. Ther. 27:219, 1980.

57. Evans, G.H., and Shand, D.G.: Disposition of propranolol. V. Drug accumulation and steady-stage concentrations during chronic oral administration in man. Clin. Pharmacol. Ther. 14:487, 1973.

58. Shand, D.G., Nukolls, E.M., and Oates, J.A.: Plasma propranolol levels in adults. Clin. Pharmacol. Ther. 11:112, 1970.

59. Briggs, W.A., Lowenthal, D.T., Cirksena, W., et al.: Propranolol in hypertensive dialysis patients: efficacy and compliance. Clin. Pharmacol. Ther. 18:606, 1975.

60. Cotham, R.H., and Shand, D.: Spuriously low plasma propranolol concentrations resulting from blood collection methods. Clin. Pharmacol. Ther. 18:535, 1975.

61. Wood, M., Shand, D.G., and Wood, A.J.J.: Altered drug binding due to sampling through heparin locks. Clin. Pharmacol. Ther. 25:255, 1979.

62. Lowenthal, D.T., Briggs, W.A., Gibson, T.P., et al.: Pharmacokinetics of oral propranolol in chronic renal disease. Clin. Pharmacol Ther. 16:761, 1974.

63. Bianchetti, G., Graziani, G., Brancaccio, D., et al.: Pharmacokinetics and effects of propranolol in terminal uraemic patients and in patients undergoing regular dialysis treatment. Clin. Pharmacokin. 1:373, 1976.

64. Lowenthal, D.T., and Mutterperl, R.: Pharmacokinetics of oral propranolol. II. The effects of chronic dosing and protein binding (abstract). Clin. Pharmacol. Ther. 19:111, 1976.

65. Lichter, M., Black, M., and Arias, I.M.: The metabolism of antipyrine in patients with chronic renal failure. J. Pharmacol. Exp. Ther. 187:612, 1973.

66. Reidenberg, M.M., Odar-Cederlof, I., von Bahr, C., et al.: Protein binding of diphenylhydantoin and desmethylimipramine in plasma from patients with poor renal function. N. Engl. J. Med. 285:264, 1971.

67. Reidenberg, M.M., Lowenthal, D.T., Briggs, W.A., et al.: Pentobarbital elimination in patients with poor renal function. Clin. Pharmacol. Ther. 20:67, 1976.

68. Walle, T., Conradi, E., Walle, K., et al.: 4-hydroxy-propranolol and its glucuronide after single and long-term doses of propranolol. Clin. Pharmacol. Ther. 27:22, 1980.

69. Schneck, D.W., Pritchard, J.F., Gibson, T.P., et al.: Effect of dose and uremeia on plasma and urine profiles of propranolol metabolites. Clin. Pharmacol. Ther. 27:744, 1980.

70. Gerhardt, R.E., Knouss, R.F., Thyrum, P.T., et al.: Quinidine excretion in aciduria and alkaluria. Ann. Intern. Med. 71:927, 1969.

71. Kessler, K.M., Lowenthal, D.T., Warner, H., et al.: Unimpaired quinidine elimination in patients with poor renal function or congestive heart failure. N. Engl. J. Med. 290:706, 1974.

72. Bellett, S., Roman, L.R., and Boza, A.: Relation between serum quinidine levels and renal function: studies in normal subjects and patients with congestive failure and renal insufficiency. Am. J. Cardiol. 27:368, 1971.

73. Drayer, D.E., Lowenthal, D.T., Restivo, K.M., et al.: Steady-state serum levels of quinidine and active metabolites in cardiac patients with varying degrees of renal function. Clin. Pharmacol. Ther. 24:31, 1978.

74. Galeazzi, R.L., Sheiner, L.B., Lockwood, T., et al.: The renal elimination of procainamide. Clin. Pharmacol. Ther. 19:55, 1976.

75. Gibson, T.P., Matusik, E.J., and Briggs, W.A.: N-acetylprocainamide levels in patients with end-stage renal failure. Clin. Pharmacol. Ther. 19:206, 1976.

76. Gibson, T.P., Lowenthal, D.T., Nelson, H.A., et al.: Elimination of procainamide in end-stage renal failure. Clin. Pharmacol. Ther. 17:321, 1975.

77. Drayer, D., Reidenberg, M.M., and Sevy, R.W.: N-acetylprocainamide: An active metabolite of procainamide. Proc. Soc. Exp. Biol. 146:358, 1974.

78. Elson, J., Strong, J.M., Lee, W.K., et al.: Antiarrhythmic potency of n-acetylprocainamide. Clin. Pharmacol. Ther. 17:134, 1975.

79. Tapia, L., Cheigh, J.S., David, D.S., et al.: Pruritus in dialysis patients treated with parenteral lidocaine. N. Engl. J. Med. 296:261, 1977.

80. Collinsworth, K.A., Kalman, S. M., and Harrison, D.C.: The clinical pharmacology of lidocaine as an antiarrhythmic drug. Circulation 50:1217, 1974.

81. Thompson, P.D., Melmon, K.L., Richardson, J.A., et al.: Lidocaine pharmacokinetics in advanced heart failure, liver disease and renal failure in humans. Ann. Intern. Med. 78:499, 1973.

82. Williams, R.L., Blaschke, T.F., Mefflin, P.J., et al.: Influence of viral hepatitis on the disposition of two compounds with high hepatic clearance: Lidocaine and indocyanine green. Clin. Pharmacol. Ther. 20:290, 1976.

83. Boyes, R.N., Scott, D.B., Jebson, P.J., et al.: Pharmacokinetics of lidocaine in man. Clin. Pharmacol. Ther. 12:105, 1971.

84. Boyes, R.N., Adams, H.J., and Duce, B.R.: Oral absorption and disposition kinetics of lidocaine hydrochloride in dogs. J. Pharm. Exp. Ther. 174:1, 1970.

85. Mason, D.T.: Disopyramide: A new agent for effective therapy of ventricular dysrhythmias. Drugs 15:329, 1978.

86. Hinderling, P.H., and Garrett, E.R.: Pharmacokinetics of the antiarrhythmic disopyramide in healthy humans. J. Pharm. Biopharm. 4:199, 1976.

87. Whiting, B., and Elliott, H.: Disopyramide in renal impairment. Lancet 2:1363, 1977.

88. Karim, A.: Disopyramide dialyzability. Lancet 2:214, 1978.

89. Boston Collaborative Drug Program: Diphenylhydantoin side effects and serum albumin levels. Clin. Pharmacol. Ther. 14:529, 1973.

90. Hahn, T.J., Hendin, B.A., Scharp, C.R., et al.: Effect of chronic anticonvulsant therapy on serum 25-hydroxycalciferol in adults. N. Engl. J. Med. 287:900, 1972.

91. Solomon, H.M., Reuh, S.D., and Spirt, N.: Interactions between digitoxin and other drugs in vitro and in vivo. Ann. N.Y. Aca. Sci. 17:362, 1971.

92. Data, J.L., Wilkinson, G.R., and Nies, A.S.: Interactions of quinidine with anticonvulsant drugs. N. Engl. J. Med. 294:699, 1976.

93. Butler, T.C.: The metabolic conversion of 5,5'diphenylhydantoin to 5-p-hydroxyphenyl-5-phenylhydantoin. J. Pharmacol. Exp. Ther. 119:1, 1957.

94. Manard, F.W.: The metabolic state of diphenylhydantoin in the dog, rat and man. J. Pharmacol. Exp. Ther. 130:275, 1960.
95. Beermann, B., Groschinsky-Grind, M., et al.: Absorption, metabolsim and excretion of hydroclorothiazide. Clin. Pharmacol. Ther. 19:531, 1976.
96. Anderson, K.V., Bretell, H.R., et al.: C^{14}-labelled hydrochlorothiazide in human beings. Arch. Intern. Med. 107:736, 1961.
97. Huang, C.M., Atkinson, A.J., et al.: Pharmacokinetics of furosemide in advanced renal failure. Clin. Pharmacol. Ther. 16:659, 1974.
98. Cutler, R.E., Forrey, A.W., Christopher, T.G., et al.: Pharmacokinetics of furosemide in normal subjects and functionally anephric patients. Clin. Pharmacol. Ther. 15:588, 1975.
99. Mitchell, J.R., and Jollows, D.J.: Progress in hepatology: metabolic activation of drugs to toxic subjects. Gastroenterology 68:392, 1975.
100. Lyons, H., Pinn, V.W., Cotrell, S., et al.: Allergic interstitial nephritis causing reversible renal failure in four patients with idiopathic nephrotic syndrome. N. Engl. J. Med. 288:124, 1973.
101. Lowenthal, D.T., Pitone, J.M., Affrime, M.B., et al.: Timolol kinetics in chronic renal insufficiency. Clin. Pharmacol. Ther. 23:606, 1978.
102. Homeida, M., Jackson, L., Roberts, C.J.: Decreased first-pass metabolism of labetalol in chronic liver disease. Br. Med., J. 2:1048, 1978.
103. Richards, D.A., Wooding, O.P., et al.: The effects of oral AH5158, a combined alpha- and beta-adrenoreceptor antagonist in healthy volunteers. Br. J. Clin. Pharm. 1:505, 1974.
104. Ohnhaus, E.E., Nuesch, E., Meier, J., et al.: Pharmacokinetics of unlabelled and ^{14}C-labelled pindolol in uremia. Eur. J. Clin. Pharm. 7:25, 1974.
105. Øie, S., and Levy, G.: Relationship between renal function and elimination kinetics of pindolol in man. Dur. J. Clin. Pharm. 9:115, 1975.
106. Tjandramaga, T.B., Thomas, J., Verbeeck, R., et al.: The effect on end-stage renal failure and hemodialysis on the elimination kinetics of sotalol. Brit. J. Clin. Pharm. 3:259, 1976.
107. Brogden, R.N., Heel, R.C., Speight, T.M., et al.: Metoprolol: A review of its pharmacological properties and therapeutic efficacy in hypertension. Drugs 14:321, 1977.
108. McAinsh, J., Holmes, B.F., Smith, S., et al.: Atenolol kinetics in renal failure. Clin. Pharmacol. Ther. 28:302, 1980.
109. Frishman, W.: Clinical pharmacology of the new beta-adrenergic blocking drugs. Part 9, Nadolol: A new long acting beta-adrenoceptor blocking drug. Am. Heart J. 99:124, 1980.
110. Herrere, J., Vukovich, R.A., and Griffith, D.L.: Elimination of nadolol by patients with renal impairment. Br. J. Clin. Pharm. 7:227S, 1979.
111. Pettinger, W.A., and Mitchell, H.C.: Clinical pharmacology of angiotensin antagonists. Fed. Proc. 35:2521, 1976.
112. Tuma, J.: Effect of saralasin on blood pressure and on hemodynamics in patients with terminal renal failure. Schweiz. Med. Wochenschr. 107:704, 1977.
113. Brunner, H.R., Wauters, J.P., McKinstry, D., et al.: Inappropriate renin secretion unmasked by captopril (SQ 14225) in hypertension in chronic renal failure. Lancet 2:704, 1978.
114. Kwan, K.C., Foltz, E.L., Breault, G.O., et al.: Pharmacokinetics of methyldopa in man. J. Pharmacol. Exp. Ther. 198:264, 1976.
115. Myhre, E., Brodwall, E.K., Stenbaek, O., et al.: Plasma turnover of methyldopa in advanced renal failure. Acta Med. Scand. 191:343, 1972.
116. An. W.Y.W, Drins, L.G., et al.: The metabolism of C^{14}-labelled alpha-

methyldopa in normal and hypertensive human subjects. Biochem. J. 129:1, 1972.

117. Yeh, B.K., Dayton, P.G., and Waters, W.C.: Removal of alpha-methyldopa in man by dialysis. Proc. Soc. Exp. Med. Biol. 135:840, 1970.

118. Dollery, C.T., Davies, D.S., Draffan, G.H., et al.: Clinical Pharmacology and pharmacokinetics of clonidine. Clin. Pharmacol. Ther. 19:11, 1976.

119. Keranen, A., Nykanen, S., Taskriness, J.: Pharmacokinetics and side effects of clonidine. Eur. J. Clin. Pharm. 13:97, 1978.

120. Fillastre, D., DuBois, D., and Brunelle, P.: Plasma half-life of C^{14}-clonidine in normal and uraemic patients, New Aspects for the treatment of arterial hypertension. Inst. Cardiovasc. Res. Univ. of Milan, Nov. 1973. Boehringer Ingelheim (Florence), pp. 81–85.

121 Hulter, H.N., Licht, J.H., Ilnicki, L.P., et al.: Clinical efficacy and pharmacokinetics of clonidine in hemodialysis and renal insufficiency. J. Lab. Clin. Med. 94:223, 1979.

122. Lowenthal, D.T., Hobbs, D. Affrime, M.B., et al.: Prazosin kinetics and effectiveness in chronic renal failure. Clin. Pharmacol. Ther. 27:779, 1980.

123. Lowenthal, D.T.: Clinical pharmacology of vasodilators. N.Y. State J. Med. 79:66, 1979.

124. Lowenthal, D.T., Onesti, G., Mutterperl, R., et al.: Long-term clinical effects, bioavailability and kinetics of minoxidil in relation to renal function. J. Clin. Pharm. 18:500, 1978.

125. Reidenberg, M.M., Drayer, D., DeMarco, A., et al.: Hydralazine elimination in man. Clin. Pharmacol. Ther. 14:970, 1978.

126. Lowenthal, D.T., Affrime, M.B., Onesti, G., et al.: Pharmacokinetics and effectiveness of antihypertensive vasodilators in chronic renal failure. Clin. Res. 26:291A, 1978.

127. Sellers, E.M., and Koch-Weser, J.: Protein-binding and vascular activity of diazoxide. N. Engl. J. Med. 281:1141, 1969.

128. Dayton, P.G., Pruitt, A.W., Faraj, B.A., et al.: Metabolism and disposition of diazoxide. Drug Metab. Dispos. 3:226, 1975.

129. O'Malley, K., Velasco, M., Pruitt, A., et al.: Decreased plasma protein binding of diazoxide in uremia. Clin. Pharmacol. Ther. 18:53, 1975.

130. McMahon, F.G.: Management of essential hypertension. Futura Publications, Mt. Kisco, N.Y., 1978, pg. 397.

131. Rahn, K.H., and Goldberg, L.I.: Comparison of antihypertensive efficacy, intestinal absorption and excretion of guanethidine in hypertensive patients. Clin. Pharmacol. Ther. 10:858, 1969.

132. Rahn, K.H.: The influence of renal function on plasma levels, urinary excretion, metabolism and antihypertensive effects of guanethidine (Ismelin) in man. Clin. Neph. 1:14, 1973.

133. Adir, J., Narang, P.K., Josselson, J., et al.: Pharmacokinetics of bretylium in renal insufficiency. N. Engl. J. Med. 300:1390, 1979.

134. Collingsworth, K.A., Strong, J.M., and Atkinson, A.J.: Pharmacokinetics and metabolism of lidocaine by patients with renal failure. Clin. Pharmacol. Ther. 18:59, 1975.

135. Lowenthal, D.T.: Pharmacokinetics of clonidine. J. Cardiovasc. Pharm. 2:529, 1980.

136. Captopril — an interesting new antihypertensive. Medical Letter: 22:39, 1980.

137. Lowenthal, D.T. and Affrime, M.B.: Pharmacology and pharmacokinetics of minoxidil. J. Cardiovasc. Pharm. 2 Suppl.: 93, 1980.

4

HEMODIALYSIS AND PERITONEAL DIALYSIS IN PATIENTS WITH CARDIAC DISEASE

ARNOLD R. EISER, M.D., AND CHARLES SWARTZ, M.D.

HEMODYNAMIC EFFECT OF HEMODIALYSIS

Clinical management of hemodialysis in patients with cardiac disease is best performed when the physician has an understanding of the hemodynamic changes which occur during dialysis. These alterations will in part depend upon the patients pretreatment state with regard to hydration, acid-base balance, electrolyte status, and cardiac rhythm. The studies of DelGreco and coworkers[1] suggest that the hemodynamic response to dialysis will differ markedly depending upon the presence or absence of congestive heart failure. They observed elevation of total peripheral resistance in both the group with congestive heart failure (CHF) and the group without; however, the elevation was more marked in those with CHF. Pretreatment cardiac output was high, normal, or low in both subjects. However, hemodialysis caused a rise in cardiac output in those with circulatory overload and a decrease in cardiac output in those without circulatory congestion.

Kim and coworkers[2] studied the hemodynamics of patients on maintenance hemodialysis (see Chapter 2). They found an elevated cardiac output related to increased heart rate without alteration of the stroke index. Total peripheral resistance was high in hypertensive uremic patients and normal or slightly decreased in normotensive uremic patients. When the anemia of uremia was corrected by blood transfusions, cardiac output decreased to normal while total peripheral resistance and mean arterial pressure increased progressively.[3] Inappropriately elevated total peripheral resistance appears to underlie the hypertension in

69

dialysis patients although the extent of vasoconstriction may be masked by the anemia.

Goss and associates[4] studied the intradialytic hemodynamic changes and found a fall in cardiac index and in stroke index occurring during dialysis with the greatest fall occurring in the first hour. Total peripheral resistance rose from a mean of 2.025 dynes/sec/cm^{-5}/m^2 to 2.968 dynes/sec/cm^{-5}/m^2. It should be noted that the patients in this study were free of hypotensive episodes during dialysis, and in fact experienced elevation of blood pressure that correlated with a rise in total peripheral resistance. Chen and others[5] found that patients who develop hypotension during dialysis had a substantially lower total peripheral resistance. They related this to blunted baroreceptor response. They found the decrease in cardiac output during dialysis equal in both the group that became hypotensive and those that did not.

Kim and associates[6] found a rapid decrease in blood volume in the first hour of dialysis which appeared to consist of rapid extravasation of the saline prime since it was not observed when a dextran prime was used. They also found that patients who became hypotensive had a lower pretreatment blood volume. Hampers and coworkers[7] found that cardiac output remained unchanged when a saline infusion during dialysis prevented weight loss. Plasma volume was reduced despite maintaining body weight constant with saline infusion.

In summary, the effect of hemodialysis on the hemodynamic parameters depends in large part on the predialysis state of hydration. In most hemodialysis treatments, a reduction in plasma volume will lead to a fall in cardiac output. However, if the patient was sufficiently hypervolemic prior to dialysis, then hemodialysis can actually increase the cardiac output by improving congestive heart failure. Whether a patient will become hypotensive on hemodialysis appears to depend on his ability to compensate for a decrease in cardiac output by increasing total peripheral resistance.

Kirsch and associates[8] found evidence of autonomic dysfunction in 6 of 8 patients who suffered from hypotensive episodes during dialysis. They observed lack of reflex tachycardia and absence of overshoot during Valsalva maneuver. In addition, the same patients manifested prolonged peroneal nerve conduction suggesting a generalized neuropathy. They further observed that hypotensive episodes could be treated successfully with norepinephrine infusion but not with volume expansion. Lilley and associates[9] also studied the mechanism of dialysis induced hypotension and described the defect as dysfunction of the afferent limb of the baroreceptor reflex. They found a correlation with lack of responsiveness to amyl nitrite vasodilatation with dialysis hypotension. They further noted that those patients with dialysis hypotension had significantly higher plasma dopamine beta-hydroxylase levels both before and after hemodialysis. They surmised that this reflected a higher resting adrenergic tone which rendered the subject less responsive to a stimulus for vasoconstriction such as hypotension. The significance of the higher beta-hydroxylase level is uncertain, however. They did not find evidence of a correlation with this defect with parameters of peripheral neuropathy. The hypotensive group had higher before and after dialysis blood pressure values and had a greater loss of plasma volume during dialysis. It would appear that a specific subset of the dialysis population has substantial impairment of reflex vasoconstriction and is thus prone to dialysis induced hypotension. Dialysis hypotension may occur either as a result of vasoconstriction dysfunction or from excessive volume depletion which results in greater reduction of the cardiac output. Table 1 summarizes the hemodynamic changes during hemodialysis.

The acid-base status of the patient is another physiologic factor which may indirectly effect hemodynamic alteration during dialysis. Carrier and associates[10] showed that at a pH of less than 7.40 or greater than 7.50 there is a general vasodilatory effect on isolated artery segments. Similar results have been found in vivo as well.[11,12] If either severe alkalemia or acidemia occurred in the course of hemodialysis, one might expect to see a fall in total peripheral resistance and resultant hypotension. In the course of hemodialysis, a respiratory alkalosis with alkalemia is the rule. Acidosis may occur in the severely ill patient where hepatic metabolism of acetate is severely impaired at the initiation of dialysis. This must be kept in mind when evaluating the patient with hypotension during dialysis.

THERAPEUTIC IMPLICATIONS FOR THE DIALYSIS PATIENT WITH CARDIAC DISEASE

The aforementioned hemodynamic alterations can guide the clinical management of the dialysis patient with cardiac disease. Those patients with heart disease and circulatory congestion derive relief from congestion and a moderate increase in cardiac output from ultrafiltration fluid removal. The patient with cardiac disease who is normovolemic or only slightly hypervolemic will need to have ultrafiltration fluid losses minimized, or cardiac output and arterial pressure may be reduced. Fluid removal can be of vital benefit to the patient with cardiac disease and renal failure but hypotension can be encountered and can result in impaired coronary perfusion. When a patient on dialysis becomes hypotensive, treatment usually consists of administration of fluids: saline, mannitol, or albumin depending upon clinical judgment of the state of hydration. At times it is more appropriate to combat hypotension with

TABLE 1. Hemodynamic changes during hemodialysis

		Cardiac index	Blood pressure	Total peripheral resistance	Heart rate	Stroke volume
Circulatory congestion present	Predialysis	L,N,H	H	H	H	N,L
	Postdialysis	↑	↓	↓	↓,O	O,↑
No circulatory congestion	Predialysis	H	N,H	N,H	H	N
	Postdialysis	↓,O	↑,O	O,↑	↑,O	↓,O
Hypotension on dialysis	Predialysis	N,H	N,H	H	H	N
	Postdialysis	↓,O	↓↓	↓↓	O	O,↓

L = low; N = normal; H = high; ↑ = increased; ↓ = decreased; O = unchanged.

vasopressor agents particularly those which increase central venous tone as well as arterial resistance. In this manner, the pathophysiologic defect in vasoconstriction can be overcome and excess fluid administration can be avoided. Metaraminol 100 mg in 500 ml of D5W can be infused slowly and has appropriate pharmacologic activity.[13] Other vasopressor agents such as L-norepinephrine and dopamine have also been used successfully.

Use of hollow fiber and parallel flow dialyzers with their low compliance offers the advantage of more predictable ultrafiltration rates and smaller extracorporeal blood volumes (see Chapter 7). Further advances in preventing hypotension during fluid removal came with the introduction of sequential hemofiltration by Ing and coworkers[14] and Bergstrom and associates.[15] This technique can be performed with standard dialysis equipment.[16] It entails the use of a negative hydrostatic pressure to cause fluid movement across the dialyzer membrane without the blood coming into contact with dialysate fluid. The absence of diffusion dialysis exerts an antihypotensive effect possibly because plasma osmolarity is not decreasing during the period of fluid loss. Chen and associates[17] studied the hemodynamic changes during hemofiltration. They found that total peripheral resistance after hemofiltration was higher for any ratio of end-diastolic left ventricular volume to total blood volume suggesting arteriolar constriction as well as venous constriction. The latter was implied by a positive correlation between cardiac output and end-diastolic volume to total blood volume ratio. The absence of any plasma osmolarity change appears to have a favorable effect on preservation of vasoconstrictive reflexes, although the manner in which diffusion dialysis interferes with vasoconstriction may be mediated by changes in pH or dialysance of vasoactive substances.

An additional advance in fluid removal techniques consists of the use of an ultrafiltration membrane with much greater water permeability such as that used in the hemofiltration technique introduced by Henderson and associates.[18] The incidence of hypotension is substantially reduced with this method. It has been suggested that such an ultrafiltration unit may be useful in the patient with pulmonary circulatory congestion even in the absence of renal failure.[19] The advantage of this procedure over sequential ultrafiltration remains to be demonstrated (see Chapter 7).

A different approach to better tolerated fluid removal in the dialysis patient with marginal cardiac reserve consists of the use of bicarbonate in lieu of the more common acetate as the dialysate buffer. Graefe and associates[20] observed better tolerated ultrafiltration in addition to less central nervous system symptoms by using a bicarbonate bath. Kirkendol and associates[21] report a negative ionotropic effect of acetate when infused into laboratory animals. This may be a factor accounting for the improved tolerance for ultrafiltration utilizing a bicarbonate bath.

In summary, hemodialysis of the cardiac patient can be guided by consideration of hemodynamic alterations. Intradialytic hypotension is the result of insufficient compensatory vasoconstriction, hence use of vasopressors can overcome the deficiency more directly than fluid administration. The newer dialysis techniques of sequential ultrafiltration and hemofiltration may permit better tolerated fluid removal by minimizing decreases in TPR (total peripheral resistance). The use of a bicarbonate bath also provides for greater cardiovascular stability possibly by eliminating a negative ionotropic effect of acetate.

ELECTROCARDIOGRAPHIC CHANGES DURING HEMODIALYSIS

Electrocardiographic changes during hemodialysis reflect the complex interaction of changing electrolyte concentrations upon a background of an already diseased myocardium (see Chapter 8). Prior to dialysis, the patient suffering from uremia will manifest an abnormal electrocardiogram;[22] most often abnormalities of the T wave, ST segment, or the QT interval are present. The T wave abnormalities generally reflect changes consistent with hyperkalemia, for example, peaking of T waves. DelGreco and Grumer[22] emphasized the fact that T wave changes of hyperkalemia may be muted by organic heart disease such as left ventricular hypertrophy with "strain" pattern as well as by digitalis effect and even myocardial infarction. Conversely, hyperkalemia may obscure electrocardiographic evidence of these organic structural abnormalities. Hence, evaluation of the electrocardiogram for evidence of organic heart disease is best made after dialysis. DelGreco and Grumer[22] also evaluated the relation between the QT interval and the plasma calcium concentration and failed to find a significant correlation. In the predialysis state, patients with normal serum calcium also manifested prolongation of the QT interval. The arrhythmogenic potential of hemodialysis was emphasized in its early use.[23,24] At least 5 percent of patients being dialyzed experience premature ventricular contractions during dialysis,[22] and this may occur independent of apparent serum electrolyte abnormalities or digoxin use.[23] Patients receiving digitalis preparations are even more likely to develop arrhythmias during dialysis. The elevation of the serum calcium concentration and decrease in the serum potassium during dialysis tends to exacerbate the electrophysiologic effects of digitalis on the myocardium. The digitalized patient may develop junctional tachycardia during dialysis which generally responds to raising the potassium concentration of the dialysate fluid.[23]

With the use of dialysate having a concentration of potassium in the 2 to 3 mEq/L range, arrhythmias are seen less frequently than when lower potassium concentrations were used.

Episodes of paroxysmal atrial tachycardia and atrial fibrillation may occur on dialysis both in the digitalized or undigitalized patient. The arrhythmias may frequently relate to excessive fluid losses and/or hypotension. They may be treated with digoxin and reduction of the ultrafiltration rate.

Matalon and coworkers[25] have called attention to the electrocardiographic artifacts that can be generated by the thrust of the blood pump during hemodialysis. This may stimulate an atrial or ventricular parasystole or may suggest dropped atrial beats. The artifactual nature of the arrhythmia can be detected by its absence in the standard lead excluding the limb with the vascular access or by turning off the pump.

Use of digoxin in dialysis patients is generally confined to those who require the drug for control of atrial arrhythmias. It is minimally removed by hemodialysis[26] and the dose must be appropriately adjusted for the level of renal impairment.[27]

DIALYSIS INDUCED HYPOXEMIA

During dialysis, the arterial partial pressure of oxygen decreases approximately 10 mm Hg.[28,29] This decrement occurs within the first 30 min of dialysis and remains fairly constant thereafter. The pathophysiology of the arterial hypoxemia has been the subject of some controversy. Early explanations of this phenomenon cited changes in pulmonary function secondary to effects of the dialysis membrane. Bischel and associates[30] suggested that microembolization producing ventilation and perfusion abnormalities resulted in an increased A-a gradient and arterial hypoxemia. They reported that use of a small pore filter in line between the dialyzer and patient abolished this change in PaO_2. Craddock and associates[28] suggested that complement mediated leukostasis during dialysis occurred in the pulmonary vasculature and resulted in acute impairment of ventilation/perfusion matching. They reported carbon monoxide diffusing capacity impaired to 70 percent and gas exchange increased in the closing volume during dialysis. They also reported pathologic evidence of intravascular pulmonary leukostasis in animals perfused with cellophane-incubated plasma. However, the pulmonary changes which they described may occur without actually altering arterial oxygen tension. Carbon monoxide diffusing capacity may be reduced without a reduction in the partial pressure of oxygen in a nonexercising subject. Likewise, the closing volume measurement may be abnormal without concomittent measurable change in arterial oxygen tension.

A subsequent explanation for this phenomenon is based on the diffusion of blood carbon dioxide across the dialyzer with ensuing loss of this gas into the dialysate. With extrapulmonary loss of CO_2, pulmonary hypoventilation would result.

Aurigemma and coworkers[29] observed that by bubbling carbon dioxide continuously into the dialysate so as to keep the partial pressure of carbon dioxide approximately 33 mm Hg, they were able to abolish the development of hypoxemia. The implication is that by preventing CO_2 loss through the dialyser, hypoventilation and subsequent hypoexemia is prevented. Shinaberger and associates[32] report that during sequential ultrafiltration where no dialysate is present, the fall in PO_2 does not occur although neutropenia does.

However, some objections have been raised to such a proposed mechanism. First, the losses of CO_2 into the dialysate are minor compared to pulmonary elimination. Second, Sherlock[33] demonstrated the fall in PaO_2 occurs in sham dialysis when blood was circulated extracorporeally through blood lines of an equivalent volume to that which would be in a dialyzer. This suggests that extracorporeal circulation itself may initiate an alteration in the ventilatory pattern that impairs ventilation/perfusion matching and the latter produces hypoxemia. Of note, in this regard is the fact that other stimuli to the respiratory center such as acidosis[31] can also prevent the fall in PaO_2.

In summary, dialysis produces a number of effects that may directly or indirectly alter pulmonary gas exchange. The occurrence of leukostasis in the pulmonary circulation may produce some alterations of pulmonary function. Diffusion of CO_2 into dialysate products is not likely to produce a significant hypoventilation reflex. Extracorporeal circulation per se may account for some alteration of ventilation thay may produce a fall in PaO_2. Other possible explanations for dialysis related hypoxemia include transudation of the saline prime sufficient to produce subclinical pulmonary congestion, or impaired ventilation/perfusion matching which occurs when the supine position is assumed. Further studies will determine the extent to which these factors contribute to this phenomenon.

In addition to arterial oxygen tension another factor that can influence adequacy of tissue oxygenation is the hemoglobin-oxygen affinity as measured by the $P_{50}O_2$. Hirszel and associates[31] observed that while $P_{50}O_2$ values decreased during dialysis, this decrement was very modest and could be attributed entirely to the Bohr effect. When the Bohr effect was eliminated, the $P_{50}O_2$ actually increased despite fall in red blood cell 2,3 diphosphoglyceric acid (2,3DPG).

The decrease in arterial oxygen tension is particularly significant in the patient suffering from cardiac disease. Occurrence of a decrease in oxygen saturation is likely to have adverse effects such as impairment of myocardial function, arrhythmia, or altered conduction. When the predialysis arterial oxygen tension is 60 mm Hg or less, the fall that can be anticipated on dialysis may result in significant oxygen desaturation. In the cardiac patient, pulmonary congestion may be responsible for arterial hypoxemia in the predialysis state. The simplest method to prevent the anticipated fall in oxygen tension is the administration of oxygen to provide a higher concentration of respired oxygen (FIO_2). Anticipation and prevention of dialysis induced hypoxemia can reduce the incidence of adverse effects during dialysis in cardiac patients.

Modifications of the dialysis procedure such as use of bicarbonate bath, avoidance of the supine position, restriction of the saline prime may also prove useful in limiting dialysis hypoxemia.

The report of Agar and others[34] suggests that some patients have a particular susceptibility to dialysis hypoxemia and display a greater drop in oxygen tension. This may be especially true in patients with sickle cell anemia when even slight hypoxemia may induce change in the erythrocyte that produces substantial impairment of pulmonary physiology.

CARDIOMYOPATHY AND DIALYSIS

Two converse relationships between dialysis and myocardial function exist. First, there may be a myocardial depressant substance in the uremic state that may be removed by dialysis. In this case, dialysis would improve myocardial function. On the other hand, a cardiomyopathy may develop during the course of maintenance hemodialysis and represent a complication of that therapy. Of course, there exist other indirect relationships between uremia, dialysis, and the function of the heart such as accelerated atherosclerosis resulting from altered lipid metabolism. These indirect relationships have been discussed in detail in previous chapters and the present discussion will be confined to the more direct interactions.

Experimental studies regarding the existence of a myocardial depressant factor in uremia have been conflicting. Scheuer and associates[35] demonstrated depressed cardiac function with an infusion of a mixture of urea, creatinine methylquanidine, and guanidinosuccinic acid. Subsequent studies in their laboratories were unable to demonstrate significant impairment of cardiac function in rats rendered uremic by subtotal nephrectomy.[36] In fact, they observed increased contractility of the myocardium in experimental acute renal failure in rats.[37] Studies in experimental chronic renal failure are also equivocal.

Clinical studies of this subject are also inconclusive. Bailey and associates[38] reported 5 patients without gross evidence of volume overload who appear to have improved cardiac function after institution of hemodialysis and considered this an instance of reversible cardiomyopathy of uremia. However, contribution of indirect factors such as hyperkalemia, acidosis, and hypertension could not be excluded. Of note is that in all their cases, the patients had clearcut evidence of pericarditis. It would be more precise to refer to this clinical entity as pancarditis rather than cardiomyopathy. Uraoka and coworkers[39] report increases in stroke work index in patients with chronic renal failure after they have undergone peritoneal dialysis. However, this increase in cardiac stroke work index was confined to those patients who had evidence of circulatory congestion. Early pathologic studies of uremic hearts in man report a myocardial lesion consisting of fatty degeneration and hazy swelling particularly of the subepicardial layers.[40,41] However, it could not be ascertained whether these were due to secondary phenomenon, for instance, hypervolemia, hyperkalemia, anemia, or acidosis.

Hence, the existence of a dialyzable myocardial depressant substance in uremia is in doubt. However, reversible myocardial depression appears to occur in uremia predominantly in association with pericarditis. Whether this is mediated by electrolyte and fluid abnormalities or is the result of a circulatory toxin remains to be established.

The converse relationship between dialysis and myocardial function to the one just discussed is the emergence of a cardiomyopathy during the course of maintenance dialysis. Drüeke and associates[42] describe some of the features and incidence of this entity. In their dialysis population, the incidence was 1.4 percent, probably greater than the prevalence of cardiomyopathy in the general population but not dramatically so. More disturbing is the report of Terman and coworkers[43] that 6 of 37 deaths in their dialysis population could be attributed to calcification of myocardial tissue. Postmortem examination in these cases revealed extensive calcification of the fibrous band of the AV node. In addition, diffuse fiber calcification was present throughout the myocardium to the extent that might produce significant impairment of contractility. Clinically, these patients have progressive stages of atrioventricular block including first degree block, interventricular conduction defect, Wenckebach phenomenon, and complete heart block. Patients also manifested elevated calcium-phosphorus product and had necropsy evidence of parathyroid hyperplasia. It would appear, then, that the greatest danger of a cardiomyopathy emerging on dialysis involves calcification of the myocardium resulting from derangement of calcium phosphate metabolism. Whether it may cause a cardiomyopathy in which the predominant feature is loss of contractility rather than deranged conduction remains to be ascertained.

Patients already afflicted with cardiac disease may be particularly susceptible to the occurrence of myocardial calcification. It is imperative that hyperphosphatemia be prevented in such patients. At times, parathyroidectomy may be necessary for the proper management of these patients' abnormal calcium metabolism.

Another feature of dialysis that may impair cardiac function is to be discussed in the next subheading. Arteriovenous fistulas created for blood access to hemodialysis are a potential iatrogenic cause of worsening cardiac function.

THE EFFECT OF ARTERIOVENOUS FISTULAS ON CARDIAC FUNCTION

Long before the advent of hemodialysis, it was known that systemic arteriovenous fistula could have adverse cardiac effect.[44,45] The presence of an arteriovenous fistula lowers peripheral resistance. Blood pressure is maintained through elevation of heart rate and blood volume expansion. Both these alterations increase cardiac work demand and when allowed to persist chronically can produce myocardial injury.

Ahearn and Maher[46] were among the first to describe this phenomenon in hemodialysis patients with Brescia-Cimino fistulas. Subsequent authors[47,48] have described this as an infrequent occurrence, but none have actually studied its incidence in a large dialysis population. The fall in heart rate during compression of the arteriovenous fistula, the Branham-Nicaladoni sign, is not invariably present in arteriovenous fistula induced high output failure. Anderson and Groce[47] reported three cases with this disorder, who did not have a positive Branham-Nicaladoni sign. They treated these patients by fixation of a Teflon band over the fistula to reduce flow. They stressed the importance of monitoring flow during the banding procedure citing the fact that flow rates are proportional to the fourth power of the vessel radius and hence a small change in the size of the anastomosis can cause a large variation in flow. They sought to maintain a flow rate between 0.4 to 0.7 L/min., although 1 L/min is probably optimal. They selected their patients on the basis of dyspnea on exertion and fatigue in the absence of other identifiable causes of worsening cardiac function. In addition, the patients demonstrated large tortuous veins with heavy thrills in their fistula site. vonBibra and associates[49] suggest that echocardiographic assessment of cardiac function may help to preselect those patients most likely to sustain symptomatic consequences of an AV fistula. They found that fistula occlusion improved parameters of cardiac contractility only in those patients who already showed evidence of impaired contractility by echocardiographic assessment prior to the fistulas.

The creation of an arteriovenous fistula for hemodialysis access may cause symptomatic cardiac failure in the patient with underlying cardiac disease. However, this appears to be an uncommon occurrence. When it does occur, it is frequently the result of aneurysmal dilatation at the anastomotic site.

When the physician encounters the dialysis patient who has worsening signs and symptoms or congestive heart failure, he may evaluate the contribution of the arteriovenous fistula by use of the Branham-Nicaladoni sign, echocardiographic assessment of cardiac function, external flow measurement, and physical signs of high arterial flow such as diffuse thrills and venous dilatation. At times, cardiac catheterization may be necessary to confirm the role of the fistula in worsening heart failure. Table 2 outlines an approach to this problem. The development of high output failure at a date far removed from the creation of the fistula suggests aneurysmal dilatation of the anastomosis. Successful treatment can be performed by banding or by complete revision of the anastomosis.

PERITONEAL DIALYSIS OF THE CARDIAC RENAL PATIENT

One of the most frequently cited advantages of peritoneal dialysis over hemodialysis is its use in patients with cardiovascular instability.[50] This premise is based on the fact that peritoneal dialysis does not require an extracorporeal blood volume or an arteriovenous blood access and the systemic electrolyte changes are less rapid. The incidence of hypotension during dialysis appears to be lower with peritoneal dialysis. In fact, in the era prior to the advent of the potent loop blocking diuretics, peritoneal dialysis was used in the treatment of pulmonary edema complicating myocardial infarction.[51,52]

However, in order to fully appreciate the application of peritoneal

TABLE 2. Evaluating the cardiac uremic patient for contribution of AV fistula to worsening heart failure

1. Exclude other causes for worsening heart function, for instance, pericarditis, volume overload, arrhythmia, worsening anemia, ischemia, hyperkalemia.
2. Evaluate for Branham-Nicaladoni sign.
3. Echocardiographic evaluation of left ventricular function—with and without graft occlusion.
4. External flow measurement. (Inaccurate if aneurysmal dilatation of anastomosis has occurred.)
5. Cardiac catheterization with and without graft occlusion failed to resolve issue, or if valvular lesion or constriction is a consideration.

dialysis in patients with cardiovascular disease, it is important to understand the hemodynamic alterations occurring during peritoneal dialysis. Of note is the fact that peritoneal dialysis has been found to be actually capable of precipitating pulmonary edema.[53-55] Swartz and others[55] found a 9.5 percent fall in the cardiac output when 2 L of dialysate fluid were infused into the peritoneum. The decrease in cardiac output could be abolished by draining the fluid out of the peritoneum. Systemic blood pressure was not changed but total peripheral resistance increased. Furthermore, the pulmonary artery pressure increased approximately 3 mm Hg. Swartz and associates also described decreased perfusion of the lower lung fields as measured by macroalbumin lung scan. Pacifico and associates[54] also observed the decreased cardiac output and elevated pulmonary artery pressure when peritoneal dialysate was infused.

It would appear then that peritoneal dialysis by causing a combined increased afterload with a reduction in cardiac output probably as a result of impaired venous return could result in the precipitation of pulmonary edema. In a patient suffering from cardiac disease, modification of the peritoneal dialysis technique may be indicated. Reduction of the volume of dialysate to one liter appears to substantially reduce the adverse effect on cardiac output. Of course, this will also reduce the dialysance of solutes. A reasonable approach in the uremic cardiac patient would be to initially start with 1 liter exchange until circulatory congestion is eliminated so that 2 liter exchanges could be performed without significant hazard.

Because of less rapid electrolyte fluxes, peritoneal dialysis is less arrhythmogenic than hemodialysis. Although instances of arrhythmias during peritoneal dialysis have been reported,[56] they have occurred in settings where other factors are more likely to be responsible for the arrhythmia. Use of peritoneal dialysis may contribute to arrhythmia indirectly, if it is used as the sole means of treatment for hyperkalemia. If serious hyperkalemia is present, rapid acting therapy such as insulin and glucose infusion must be utilized in conjunction with the peritoneal dialysis.

Peritoneal dialysis is a dehydrating procedure. Usually this is beneficial for the cardiac patient. Although, if the patient is in the euhydrated state prior to initiation of dialysis, and in addition, has impaired thirst mechanism, hypovolemia and hypotension may occur unless adequate fluid replacement is provided.

The recent experience with chronic maintenance peritoneal dialysis appears to indicate that this is a suitable alternative to hemodialysis.[57,58] Of note, however, is the report of Roxe[57] which suggests that episodes of circulatory congestion may be more frequent with maintenance peritoneal dialysis. In summary then, it is unclear at this point whether peritoneal dialysis offers a clearcut advantage to hemodialysis in the patient suffering from cardiovascular disease, and it would appear that selection of the appropriate modality will have to be individualized.

REFERENCES

1. DelGreco, F., Simon, N., Rogusku, J., et al.: Hemodynamic studies in chronic uremia. Circulation 40:87, 1969.
2. Kim, K.E., Onesti, G., and Swartz, C.: Hemodynamics of hypertension in uremia. Kid. Int. 8 (5):155, 1975.
3. Neff, J.S., Kim, K.E., Persoff, M., et al.: Circulation 43:876, 1971.
4. Goss, J.E., Alfrey, A.C., Vogel, J.H., et al.: Hemodynamic changes during hemodialysis. Trans. Amer. Soc. Artif. Intern. Organs 13:68, 1967.
5. Chen, W-T, Chaignon, M., Taruzi, R.C., et al.: Hemodynamics of post-dialysis hypotension. Abstr. Amer. Soc. Neph. 1977, p. 41A.
6. Kim, K.E., Neff, M., Cohen, B., et al.: Blood volume changes and hypotension during dialysis. Trans. Amer. Soc. Artif. Intern. Organs 16:508, 1970.
7. Hampers, C.L., Skillman, J.J., Lyons, J.H., et al.: Hemodynamic evaluation of bilateral nephrectomy and hemodialysis in hypertensive men. Circulation 35:272, 1967.
8. Kirsch, E.S., Kronfield, J.S., Unger, A., et al.: Autonomic insufficiency in uremia as a cause of hemodialysis induced hypotension. N. Engl. J. Med. 290:650, 1974.
9. Lilley, J.J., Golden, J., and Stone, R.A.: Adrenergic regulation of blood pressure in chronic renal failure. J. Clin. Invest. 57:1190, 1976.
10. Carrier, O., Cowsert, M., Hancock, J., et al.: Effect of hydrogen ion changes on vascular resistance in isolated artery segments. Am. J. Physiol. 207:168, 1964.
11. Deal, C.P., and Green, H.D.: Effects of pH on blood flow and peripheral resistance in muscular and cutaneous vascular beds in the hind limb of the pentobarbitalized dog. Circ. Res. 2:148, 1954.
12. Kester, N.C., Richardson, and Green, H.D.: Effect of controlled hydrogen-ion concentration on peripheral vascular tone and blood flow in innervated hind leg of the dog. Am. J. Physiol. 169:678, 1952.
13. Hampers, C.L., Schupak, E., Lowrie, E.G., et al.: Long Term Hemodialysis. Grune & Stratton, New York, 1973, pg. 86.
14. Ing, T.S., Ashback, D.L., Kanter, A., et al.: Fluid removal with negative-pressure hydrostatic ultrafiltration using a partial vacuum. Nephron 14:451, 1975.
15. Bergstrom, J., Asaba, H., Furst, P., et al.: Dialysis, ultrafiltration and blood pressure. Proc. Eur. Dial. Transplant Assoc. 13:293, 1976.
16. Shinaberger, J.H., Brantbar, N., Miller, J.H., et al.: Successful application of sequential hemofiltration followed by diffusion dialysis with standard dialysis equipment. Trans. Am. Soc. Artif. Intern. Organs 24:677, 1978.
17. Chen, W.T., Chaignon, M., Omvik, P., et al.: Hemodynamic studies in chronic hemodialysis patients with hemofiltration/ultrafiltration. Trans. Am. Soc. Artif. Intern. Organs 24:682, 1978.
18. Henderson, L.W., Besarab, A., and Michaels, A.: Blood purification by ultrafiltration and fluid replacement (diafiltration). Trans. Amer. Soc. Artif. Intern. Organs 13:216, 1967.

19. Silverstein, M.E., Ford, C.A., Lysaght, M.J., et al.: Treatment of severe fluid overload by ultrafiltration. N. Engl. J. Med. 291:747, 1974.

20. Graefe, U., Milutinovich, J., Foltette, W.C., et al.: Less dialysis-induced morbidity and vascular instability with bicarbonate in dialysate. Ann. Intern. Med. 88:332, 1978.

21. Kirkendol, P.L., and Devia, C.J.: The comparison of the cardiovascular effects produced by infusions of sodium bicarbonate and sodium acetate in dogs. Abstr. Amer. Soc. Neph. 1978, p. 44A.

22. DelGreco, F., and Grumer, H.: Electrolyte and electrocardiographic changes in the course of hemodialysis. Am. J. Cardiol. 9:43, 1962.

23. Rubin, A.L., Lubash, G.D., Cohen, B.D., et al.: Electrocardiographic changes during hemodialysis with the artificial kidney. Circulation, 43:227, 1958.

24. Kohn, R.M., and Kiley, J.E.: Electrocardiographic changes during hemodialysis with observations on contributions of electrolyte disturbances to digitalis toxicity. Ann. Intern. Med., 39:38, 1953.

25. Matalon, R., Nidus, B.D., and Eisinger, R.P.: Pseudoarrhythmias during hemodialysis. N. Engl. J. Med. 278:1439, 1968.

26. Ackerman, G.L., Doherty, J.E., and Flanigan, W.J.: Peritoneal dialysis and hemodialysis of tritiated digoxin. Ann. Intern. Med. 67:718, 1967.

27. Gault, M.H., Jeffrey, J.R., Chirito, E., et al.: Studies of digoxin dosage, kinetics, and serum concentrations in renal failure and review of the literature. Nephron 17:161, 1976.

28. Craddock, P.R., Fehr, J., Brigham, K.L., et al.: Complement and leukocyte-mediated pulmonary dysfunction in hemodialysis. N. Engl. J. Med. 296:769, 1977.

29. Aurigemma, N.M., Feldman, N.T., Gottlieb, M., et al.: Arterial oxygenation during hemodialysis. N. Engl. J. Med. 297:871, 1977.

30. Bischel, M.D., Scoles, B.G., and Mohler, T.G.: Evidence for pulmonary microembolization during hemodialysis. Chest 67:335, 1975.

31. Hirszel, P., Maher, J.F., Tempel, G.E., et al.: Effect of hemodialysis on factors influencing oxygen transport. J. Lab. Clin. Med. 85:978, 1975.

32. Shinaberger, J.H., Brautbar, N., Miller, J.H., et al.: Clinical and physiological studies of sequential ultrafiltration—diffusion dialysis. Abstr. Amer. Soc. Neph. 1978, p. 51A.

33. Sherlock, J.: Symposia on acid-base changes during dialysis. Trans. Amer. Soc. Artif. Intern. Organs 23:406, 1977.

34. Agar, J.W., Hull, J.D., Kaplan, M., et al.: Acute cardiopulmonary decompensation and complement activation during hemodialysis. Ann. Intern. Med. 90:792, 1979.

35. Scheuer, J., and Stezoski, S.W.: The effects of uremic compounds on cardiac function and metabolism. J. Mol. Cell. Card. 5:287, 1973.

36. Scheuer, J., Mivatpumin, T., and Yipintsoi, T.: Effects of moderate uremia on cardiac contractile response. Proc. Soc. Exp. Bio. Med. 150:471, 1975.

37. Mivatpumin, T., Yipintsoi, T., and Penpargkul, S.: Increased cardiac contractility in acute uremia: interrelations with hypertension. Am. J. Physiol. 229:501, 1975.

38. Bailey, G.L., Hampers, C.L., and Merill, J.P.: Reversible cardiomyopathy in uremia. Trans. Am. Soc. Artif. Int. Organs 13:263, 1967.

39. Uraoka, P., Sugimoto, T., Inaska, T., et al.: Changes of cardiac performance in renal failure. Jap. Heart J. 26:489, 1975.

40. Gouley, B.A.: The myocardial degeneration associated with uremia. Am. J. Med. Sci. 200:39, 1940.

41. Soloman, C., Roberts, J.E., and Lisa, J.R.: The heart in uremia. Am. J. Pathol. 18:729, 1942.
42. Drüeke, T., LePailleru, C., Meilhae, B., et al.: Congestive cardiomyopathy in uremic patients on long term haemodialysis. Br. Med. J. 1:350, 1977.
43. Terman, D.S., Alfrey, A.C., Hammond, W.D., et al.: Cardiac calcification in uremia. Am. J. Med. 50:744, 1971.
44. Warren, J.V., Nickerson, J.G., and Eklin, D.C.: The cardiac output in patients with arteriovenous fistula. J. Clin. Invest. 30:210, 1951.
45. Muenster, J.J., Graettinger, J.S., and Campbell, J.A.: Correlation of clinical and hemodynamic findings in patients with systemic arteriovenous fistulas. Circulation 20:1079, 1959.
46. Ahearn, D.J., and Maher, J.F.: Heart failure as a complication of hemodialysis arteriovenous fistula. Ann. Intern. Med. 77:201, 1972.
47. Anderson, C.B., and Groce, M.A.: Banding of arteriovenous dialysis fistulas to correct high-output cardiac failure. Surgery 78:552, 1975.
48. Draur, R.A.: Heart failure and dialysis fistulas. Ann. Intern. Med. 79:765, 1973.
49. vonBibra, H., Castro., L., Autenrieth, G., et al.: The effect of arteriovenous shunts on cardiac function in renal dialysis patients—an echocardiographic evaluation. Clin. Nephrol 9:205, 1978.
50. Tenckhoff, H.: Chronic Peritoneal Dialysis Manual. University of Washington Press, Seattle, 1974, p. 13.
51. Mailloux, L.U., Swartz, C.D., Onesti, G., et al.: Peritoneal dialysis for refractory congestive heart failure. JAMA 199:873, 1967.
52. Chopra, M.P., Gulati, R.B., Portal, R.W., et al.: Peritoneal dialysis for pulmonary edema after acute myocardial infarction. Br. Med. J. 3:77, 1970.
53. Maher, J.F., and Schreiner, G.E.: Hazards and complication of dialysis. N. Engl. J. Med. 273:370, 1965.
54. Pacifico, A.D., Lasker, N., Frank, M.L., et al.: Cardiovascular function in peritoneal dialysis. Trans. Amer. Soc. Artif. Int. Organs 11:86, 1965.
55. Swartz, C., Onesti, G., Mailloux, L., et al.: The acute hemodynamic and pulmonary effects of peritoneal dialysis. Trans. Amer. Soc. Artif. Int. Organs 15:367, 1969.
56. Rutsky, E.A.: Bradycardia rhythms during peritoneal dialysis. Arch. Intern. Med. 128:445, 1971.
57. Roxe, D.M.: Comparisons of maintenance peritoneal and hemodialysis. Dialysis Transpl. 7:792, 1978.
58. Blumenkrantz, M.J.: Controlled evaluation of maintenance peritoneal dialysis. Dialysis Transpl. 7:797, 1978.

5

PERICARDIAL DISEASE IN CHRONIC RENAL FAILURE

MORRIS N. KOTLER, M.D., F.R.C.P., AND WAYNE R. PARRY

Richard Bright[1] described uremic pericarditis in 1836. Before the advent of dialysis and transplantation, pericarditis was considered a terminal event in patients with chronic renal disease. With the widespread use of chronic hemodialysis, uremic pericarditis has assumed an important role, since it is one of the complications of chronic renal failure that may respond to treatment.

INCIDENCE

The incidence of uremic pericarditis has been reported to vary between 14 and 20 percent in patients undergoing dialysis.[2-5] Prior to 1960 when chronic hemodialysis was introduced, Wacker and Merrill[6] reported a 50 percent incidence of pericarditis in patients with chronic renal failure. The incidence of pericarditis in the undialyzed patient has decreased presumably because of improved conservative management by diet therapy and earlier selection for chronic hemodialysis or transplantation.[7] However, the incidence of pericarditis in the dialyzed patient is now higher than that in the untreated patient.

PHYSIOLOGY OF THE PERICARDIUM

Several functions have been ascribed to the pericardium. These include:
1. Lubrication. The double layered pericardium with its potential space is filled with fluid which acts as a lubricant so that the heart can undergo motion without friction or damage.[8]

2. Protection from infection. Lymphatic drainage from the myocardium accumulates on the surface of the epicardium which is then drained into the lymphatic system.[9] The active turnover of lymph is regarded as a defense mechanism and protects the heart from infection via contiguous structures.

3. Equalization of gravitational forces.[10] The heart can significantly shift with alterations in posture. One of the functions of the pericardium is to limit the extent of mobility of the heart within the thorax.

4. Restraining effect of the pericardium. Recent studies have focused on the importance of the pericardium in limiting cardiac dilatation.[11-13] The role of the pericardium as a determinant of the relationship between the diastolic pressure and dimension of the left and right ventricle has also been studied. Normal intrapericardial pressure is subatmospheric and declines during inspiration. Intrapericardial pressure rises when cardiac volume is increased and falls when intracardiac volume decreases. Pericardial pressure is determined by the compliance characteristics of the pericardium and total intrapericardial volume.[8] This volume consists of the pericardial fluid and heart volumes. In experimental animal models, intracardiac chambers dilate acutely when hypervolemia is present.[13] The degree of dilatation is eventually limited by the stiff pericardium. Left ventricular diastolic pressure elevation is thus influenced by the other dilated intrapericardial structures as well as the restraining influence of the pericardium itself.[13] Following removal of the pericardium, the major determinant of ventricular diastolic pressure is the dimension of the left ventricle.[13]

PATHOGENESIS

No specific etiologic factor can be implicated as a cause of uremic pericarditis. There is no absolute correlation between the development of pericarditis and the blood urea levels.

Current consensus is that a serositis, coupled with the hemorrhagic diathesis (presumably the result of a platelet defect and/or decreased fibrinolytic activity), is the initiating event in uremic pericarditis.[7,60] Continued trauma to the inflamed pericardial surfaces by continued contraction and relaxation of the myocardium perpetuates this process.[7] Why some patients with uremic pericarditis do not resolve following control of uremia and why some stable patients develop pericarditis during chronic hemodialysis is unexplained. Additional factors implicated in the development of pericarditis in the dialyzed patient include: inadequate dialysis, infection, surgical procedures, duration of dialysis, hypercalcemia, and heparin therapy. Increasing dialysis frequency from two to three times weekly has decreased the influence of pericarditis. In addition, intensification of dialysis has been associated with resolution of pericarditis in approximately 30 percent of cases without anti-inflammatory drugs or surgical interventions.[2,5] These findings have not been universally accepted and other investigators have observed re-peated episodes of pericarditis in stable patients who were being di-alyzed on a three times a week basis.[14] The infective theory with isolation of bacteria has been unconvincing in the majority of instances but on oc-casion isolated cases of bacterial pericarditis have been reported after severe transplant rejection[15] or in severely debilitated patients with generalized sepsis.[16] Cytomegalovirus (CMV) has been implicated as a causative agent in one study.[17]

Uncomplicated surgical procedures may produce a catabolic state which in turn will increase dialysis requirements.[7] The majority of pa-tients in our institution who have developed uremic pericarditis have *not* undergone a recent surgical procedure. There is no correlation between the duration of hemodialysis and the development of pericarditis.[7] Hypercalcemia or secondary hyperparathyroidism have been implicated as causative factors, but many patients with severe hyperparathyroidism requiring parathyroidectomy have not developed pericarditis.[7] Most in-vestigators believe that heparin is not the initiating factor but that it may perpetuate the inflammatory process by causing repeated bleeding from the inflamed pericardial surfaces.[7]

PATHOLOGY

The pathologic spectrum of uremic pericarditis is variable. Initially, an aseptic inflammatory process with fibrin formation has been described. Patients with untreated uremia at autopsy may demonstrate the char-acteristic "bread and butter" appearance of the pericardium. In more severe cases, extensive thickening of both layers of the pericardium with areas of hemorrhage may be found. Fibrinous adhesions between the visceral pericardium and epicardium are common. Pericardial fluid which is frequently found may be serous, serosanguineous, or frankly hemorrhagic. In subacute constrictive pericarditis, the inflammatory pro-cess may be more profound and pericardial fibrosis may be marked.[14] In chronic constrictive pericarditis, both layers of the pericardium are markedly thickened by fibrosis and may be adherent to each other and to the underlying epicardium. Calcification does not occur in constrictive pericarditis secondary to uremia.[7] In some patients, extension of the in-flammatory process to the underlying myocardium may occur.[2] The in-flammatory process with its extension may be responsible for the myocardiopathy that has been reported in patients with pericarditis from other causes.[2,18,19]

CLINICAL FEATURES

The majority of patients with uremic pericarditis develop pericardial effusion; a small percentage going on to tamponade. However, in some patients pericarditis may occur without evidence of pericardial effusion. Chest pain is a frequent manifestation occurring in 63 to 71 percent of patients[2-4] (Table 1). The pain may be severe and may resemble the pain of myocardial infarction. At times, the severity, location, and radiation of pain in acute pericarditis is extremely variable. The precordial pain may be abrupt and sharp with a wide area of radiation to the neck, back, left shoulder, and occasionally to the arm. The pleura also may be involved in the inflammatory process and frequently a sharp pleuritic type of pain may occur during respiration. Why some patients with uremic pericarditis do not develop chest pain is unknown.[7] Possible explanations for this phenomenon include absence of inflammatory process of the small lower parietal pain sensitive area of the pericardium, or the pain threshold may not be reached because the inflammation is mild or slowly progressing.[20] The pain is commonly increased by motion such as rotation of the trunk and deep breathing or bending. Swallowing, coughing, or yawning can aggravate the pain. The pain may be accentuated in the lying position and relieved by sitting up or leaning forward. A pericardial friction rub is present in over 90 percent of cases. The friction rub may be transitory or absent in 5 to 8 percent of cases. A friction rub can occur in the presence of moderate to large pericardial effusion as well as in tamponade.[20] Although the friction rub can change in character from minute

TABLE 1. Clinical features of uremic pericarditis

Author (%) Frequency	Comty et al[2] 1971	Ribot et al[3] 1974	Silverberg et al[4] 1977
Feature			
Pain	64	71	63
Pericardial friction rub	92	95	91
Fever	96	76	79
Leukocytosis	71	62	35
Cardiac arrhythmia	28	19	23
Hypotension	56	—	—
Hepatomegaly	60	—	—
Elevated venous pressure	71	—	—
Abnormal ECG	88	—	92
Cardiomegaly	92	100	—

to minute, a classic superficial quality that is described as scratchy or grating is frequently audible. The patient should be examined in various positions such as lying, sitting, or leaning forward. The rub is frequently accentuated during inspiration. The number of components of the friction rub and the intensity of each relate to the force of the cardiac motion response for that component. The ventricular systolic component is the loudest, longest, and best heard and occurs in practically all cases.[21] The presystolic component is synchronous with atrial contraction and heard in approximately 70 percent of cases.[21] The protodiastolic component is the least constant of the three and is synchronous with rapid diastolic filling. It occurs in approximately 60 percent of cases.[21] Triphasic rubs may be heard in 50 percent of cases and the true biphasic rub in 25 percent of patients. Frequently the protodiastolic and presystolic phases cannot be separated, resulting in the apparent biphasic "to and fro" quality.[21]

Additional findings that are frequently present at the time of presentation include fever, leukocytosis, and cardiomegaly.[2-4] Pericarditis should be considered in the differential diagnosis in any patient with advanced chronic renal failure who demonstrates progressive right heart failure associated with increasing heart size. These patients frequently have concomitant hypertension, fluid overload, and primary myocardial disease, all complicating the differential diagnosis of progressive heart failure.

A fall in blood pressure or hypotension, per se, in patients with chronic renal failure who are undergoing hemodialysis should alert the clinician to the possibility of massive pericardial effusion or cardiac tamponade. Hypotension during dialysis may also occur as a result of bacteremia, extracellular volume depletion, pyrogen reaction, arrhythmias, and progressively severe left ventricular dysfunction secondary to underlying coronary artery disease[7] (see Chapter 11). In rapidly accumulating effusions, profound hypotension and a shock-like state may occur. In more slowly accumulating effusions, the diagnosis of cardiac tamponade may be easily overlooked. Neck vein engorgement, tachycardia, and a diminished pulse pressure are characteristic. Pulsus paradoxus may be present. Pulsus paradoxus is a misnomer because it is in point of fact an exaggeration of a normal response.[22] During quiet breathing in a normal healthy individual, inspiratory decrease in arterial pressure does not exceed 10 mm Hg and usually averages 3 to 5 mm Hg. Many factors contribute to the production of the normal inspiratory decline in arterial blood pressure. These include transmission of the inspiratory decline in intrathoracic pressure to the heart and aorta, and a transit delay in the lungs of the normal inspiratory increase in right ventricular stroke volume. The augmented right ventricular output associated with inspiration is not discernable in the arterial system until the succeeding expiration, and, therefore, arterial pressure appears to fall slightly during inspiration. Changes in heart rate and inspiratory increase in right ventricular filling with raised intrapericardial pressure resulting in left ventricular compression and autonomic reflex activity may contribute to the net respiratory change in arterial pressure. Pulsus paradoxus is defined as an abnormal inspiratory decline in blood pressure, usually greater than 10 mm Hg.[23,24] The inspiratory decline in systolic blood pressure results in a striking inspiratory decrease in the arterial pulse pressure (Fig. 1). With extreme cardiac tamponade and in the presence of severe hypotension[7] and severe left ventricular failure,[25] pulsus paradoxus may not be appreciated. The most reliable method of measuring pulsus paradoxus is by the cuff method.[24] The cuff is deflated slowly and the upper recording is measured by the pressure reading at which systolic sounds are heard only in expiration. The lower recording is measured by the pressure reading at which sounds are heard throughout the respiratory cycle. The difference between the two readings is the inspiratory decrease in arterial pressure or pulsus paradoxus. Several theories have been advanced but probably there is no single explanation for the occurrence of pulsus paradoxus in cardiac tamponade.[24]

Several factors combine to reduce the arterial pressure during inspiration. At the beginning of inspiration venous return to the right atrium in-

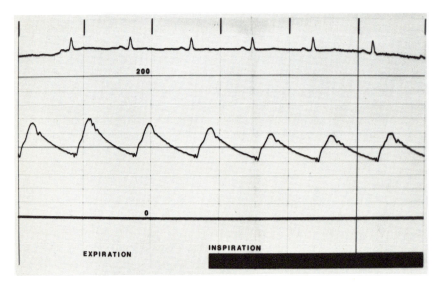

FIGURE 1. Pulsus paradoxus recorded in a patient with chronic renal failure and a large pericardial effusion. Note the characteristic inspiratory decline of arterial pressure from 140 mm Hg to 116 mm Hg—paradoxus of 24 mm Hg.

creases. The augmentation in venous return is followed by an increase in right ventricular stroke volume. In the presence of cardiac tamponade, inspiration produces a small but definite increase in transmural pericardial pressure (pericardial pressure minus pleural pressure) which may cause some degree of left ventricular compression. With hemodynamically significant pericardial effusion, inspiratory right ventricular volume is increased less than normal because of impaired filling, but the increased capacity of the pulmonary vascular bed with inspiration is not impaired.[22] The combined effect of the increased capacity of the pulmonary vascular bed with inspiration plus the increased stretch of the pericardium and the raised intrapericardial pressure result in depression of left ventricular stroke volume and greater than normal decline of systolic pressure on inspiration.[22] Ewart's sign may be present and is characterized by an area of dullness and bronchial breathing at the left lung base. The sign usually results from lung compression due to a retrodisplaced heart and posterior bulging of the lateral portion of the pericardium.

The electrocardiogram is of minimal value in the diagnosis of uremic pericarditis. In one study only 5 percent of the electrocardiograms showed the ST segment elevations regarded as characteristic of pericarditis.[4] Nonspecific ST and T wave changes and left ventricular hypertrophy patterns may be frequently recorded.[4] Cardiac arrythmias, especially atrial flutter or fibrillation, may be the presenting feature of uremic pericarditis in some patients.[2-5] Atrial arrythmias may be frequently recorded varying from 19 to 28 percent.[2-4] Silverberg and colleagues[4] reported that reticulocyte counts were greater than 6 percent in 62 percent of patients with chronic renal failure and pericarditis who were undergoing dialysis. In 24 percent of the patients, reticulocyte counts were greater than 10 percent. The reticulocyte counts were significantly higher in patients with uremic pericarditis than in patients without pericarditis. The exact mechanism of the high reticulocyte count remains unclear but may be due to hemorrhage into the pericardial sac, red blood cell breakdown, and subsequent reutilization of the iron in erythropoiesis.[4]

Pleural effusion, unilateral or bilateral, on x-ray is common in uremic pericarditis and may be a manifestation of "uremic pleural effusion."[4] Fluid overload and/or associated congestive heart failure may be partially responsible for pleural effusions as well. The heart is enlarged on x-ray in over 90 percent of patients with uremic pericardial effusions.[2] Increasing heart size on serial chest x-ray especially in the absence of heart failure should alert the clinician to the possibility of uremic pericardial effusion.

DIAGNOSIS

The echocardiogram is the simplest, safest, and probably the most accurate method of diagnosing pericardial fluid (and for assessing left ventricular function in chronic uremia[61]). In our institution, echocardiography has replaced intravenous arteriography and pericardial scanning in the diagnosis of pericardial effusion. Several studies have attested to the value of echocardiography in the diagnosis of pericardial effusion.[26-28]

Technique is of paramount importance in the echocardiographic diagnosis of pericardial effusion. With the patient in the recumbent position and the trunk elevated 20 to 30 degrees, the transducer is placed in the third, fourth, or fifth intercostal space. The mitral valve is identified and the transducer is angulated in an inferior and lateral direction to record echoes of the left ventricular posterior wall at the chordae tendineae level. Clear visualization of the anterior right ventricular wall and septum can usually be accomplished by careful adjustments of reject, gain intensity, and damping controls. With regard to the left ventricular posterior wall, all the components must be identified, namely, endocardium, myocardium, epicardium, and pericardium (Fig. 2). During the actual recording of the left ventricular posterior wall, the intensity of the echograph is reduced (gain is decreased) so that the dominant strong posterior pericardial echo which moves anteriorily during systole is recorded (Fig. 2).

In patients with pericardial effusions, fluid first appears posteriorly in the dependent portion of the pericardial cavity. Therefore, small pericardial effusions can be recognized by minimal separation of the left ventricular posterior wall epicardial echo from the relatively stationary pericardial echo (Fig. 2A). Small effusions result in separation through systole and part of diastole. With increasing accumulation of fluid the posterior echo free space becomes evident throughout the entire cardiac cycle. With larger effusions the posterior echo free space widens, and fluid appears anteriorly as an anterior echo free space (Fig. 2B). The detection of anterior echo free spaces without the detection of posterior pericardial effusion may represent epicardial fat rather than fluid. In the majority of instances pericardial fluid lying between the posterior epicardium and the pericardium disappears at the atrioventricular junction as the ultrasonic beam is angulated toward the left atrium. However, in large pericardial effusions fluid may be detected behind the left atrium which represents accumulation of fluid in the oblique sinus of the pericardium.[27,28]

In patients with very large pericardial effusions, a swinging motion of the heart can occur. The anterior wall motion may become more striking than that of the posterior heart wall. In this type of situation the posterior

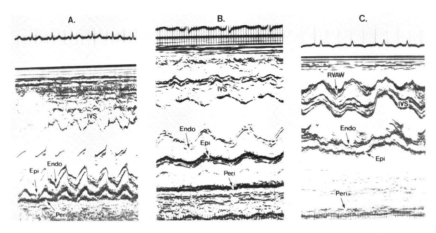

FIGURE 2. M-mode echocardiograms in 3 patients with chronic renal failure. A. Small posterior pericardial effusion with separation of epicardium (Epi) from stationary pericardium (Peri). With excessive damping (left hand side), each component of the left ventricular posterior wall and echo free space representing pericardial fluid is seen. B. Moderate pericardial effusion. A moderate echo free space separates epicardium and stationary pericardium. Concentric hypertrophy is present. C. Massive pericardial effusion with large anterior and posterior echo free spaces. There is a swinging motion of the pericardium and decrease in right ventricular cavity size. IVS = septum; Endo = endocardium; RVAW = right ventricular anterior wall.

cardiac structures may not be recorded because the anterior right ventricular wall becomes a strong reflector of ultrasound and diminishes the energy available for deeper penetration (Fig. 3). The excessive rotation of the heart recorded in the *swinging heart syndrome* occurs as a result of the absence of the restraining function of the pericardium. As a consequence of the excessive swinging of the heart, abnormal motion of all the intracardiac valves and the septum has been noted.[29,30] When swinging becomes so excessive that the heart does not return to its original position before the next electrical depolarization, the phenomenon of *electrical alternans* takes place[31,32] (Fig. 3).

Accurate quantitation of pericardial effusions by echocardiography is not reliable. However, using the criteria outlined above, semiquantitative assessments can be made, that is, minimal, small, moderate, large and massive effusions. Horowitz and associates[26] compared echocardiographic criteria for pericardial effusions with the amount of pericardial effusion found in patients undergoing cardiac surgery. They established the lower limit of sensitivity of a technically optimal, properly interpreted echocardiogram as 15 to 20 ml.[26] Despite the simplicity

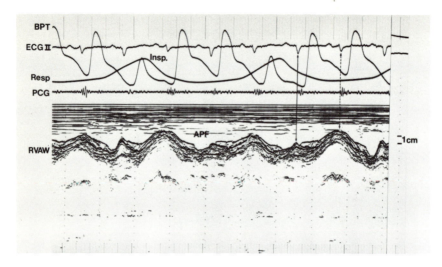

FIGURE 3. Massive pericardial effusion with large anterior echo free space and "swinging heart syndrome." At the time of the first QRS complex, the anterior wall of the right ventricle is in its most anterior location closest to the chest wall. Following this, the anterior wall moves posteriorly and does not return to its original anterior position with the next electrical depolarization. With the third QRS complex, the anterior wall of the right ventricle moves more anteriorly to the chest wall. Note pulsus and electrical alternans. Posterior lying structures were not adequately recorded presumably because the ultrasound beam strongly reflects from the anterior right ventricular wall with inability of the sound wave to penetrate deeper structures. BPT = brachial pulse tracing; Resp = respiration; PCG = phonocardiogram; RVAW = right ventricular anterior wall; APF = anterior pericardial fluid.

of echocardiography in establishing the diagnosis of pericardial effusion there are pitfalls with regard to technique and interpretation of echocardiograms.[33] Excessively low gain settings may result in incomplete identification of the various components of the left ventricular posterior wall; too high gain settings can result in excessive echoes thus obscuring the recognition of an echo free space. If the transducer is angulated too far medially, an echo free space behind the posterior wall can be recorded. Frequently the mitral annulus recorded in this position may be mistaken for the left ventricular posterior wall. Echo free spaces behind the medial aspect of the posterior wall may be recorded. This may occur as a result of the coronary sinus, descending aorta, or other posterior mediastinal structures. Calcified mitral annulus, which is a frequent finding in chronic renal failure,[34] may be mistaken for the left ventricular posterior wall and the echo free space behind the annulus may be mistaken for pericardial fluid. Echo free spaces behind the posterior left ventricular wall can occur in pleural effusions or pulmonary infiltrates.

Two dimensional echocardiography and slow M-mode scanning are useful in detecting accumulations of pericardial fluid at the apex. Additional cross sectional images obtained at various planes of the left ventricle may be confirmatory in diagnosing pericardial effusion. Vigorous inward motion of the myocardium with relative stationary pericardium separated by an echo free space is characteristic.

Echocardiographic recognition of tamponade has been described by several investigators,[35,36] although in our experience cardiac tamponade remains a clinical syndrome. The swinging heart syndrome with electrical or pulsus alternans should alert the clinician to the possibility of tamponade.

Changes in mitral valve motion and chamber dimensions have been reported to be indicative of tamponade. Decreased excursion of the mitral valve with diminished EF slope during inspiration was noted.[35] The inspiratory alteration in mitral valve motion was accompanied by an increase in right ventricular dimensions and a reciprocal decrease in left ventricular dimensions.[35] The variation in chamber dimensions with respiration may be associated with pulsus paradoxus that is commonly found in these patients. Additional less specific findings include a notch on the epicardial surface of the right ventricle occurring during the isometric contraction phase of the cardiac cycle[36] and coarse oscillations of the left ventricular posterior wall. Recently, Schiller and Botvinick[37] described right ventricular compression as a sign of cardiac tamponade in 17 patients with pericardial effusion. The right ventricular minor axis at end-diastole and at expiration measured 7 ± 2 mm or less. We have found this sign useful in the diagnosis of pericardial tamponade especially by two dimensional echocardiography (Fig. 4). However, its absence does not preclude cardiac tamponade.

In our institution, we have found that echocardiography is particularly useful in differentiating pericardial effusion from other commonly observed abnormalities in patients with chronic renal failure (Figs. 5–7). One hundred and ten patients with chronic renal failure were studied by echocardiography.[38] Pericardial effusion was the most frequent echocardiographic finding accounting for 55 percent of patients (Fig. 5). Concentric hypertrophy was present in 36 percent of patients (Fig. 6) and left ventricular enlargement in 40 percent.

In addition, three distinct echocardiographic patterns of left ventricular function were observed: the hyperkinetic pattern, the left ventricular dilatation pattern, and the cardiomyopathy pattern (Fig. 7). The

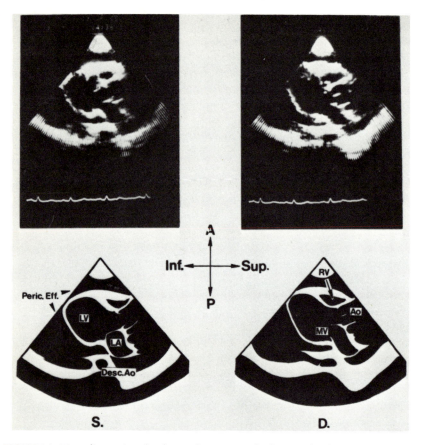

FIGURE 4. Two dimensional echocardiogram in the longitudinal view in a patient with chronic renal failure and pericardial tamponade. There is a massive effusion which surrounds the heart; more prominent at the apex. The right ventricular cavity is compressed at the apex and is diminished in size at the outflow tract. An idealized diagram of each frame (below) is presented in systole (S) and diastole (D). Ao = aorta; Desc. = descending; LA = left atrium; LV = left ventricle; MV = mitral valve; Peric. Eff. = pericardial effusion; RV = right ventricle.

latter pattern was seen in 25 percent of patients. Hypokinesis of the septum and left ventricular posterior wall were characteristic features (Fig. 7). In addition to left ventricular cavity enlargement, abnormal mitral valve closure was present in some patients. Additional echocardiographic findings included: asymmetric septal hypertrophy, aortic sclerosis, and mitral annular calcification. Thus, echocardiography is extremely helpful in differentiating pericardial effusion from increasing

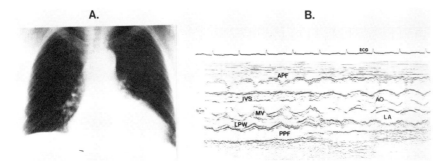

FIGURE 5. A, X-ray in a patient with chronic renal failure and an enlarged heart. B, Same patient demonstrating a moderate pericardial effusion with anterior and posterior echo free space. Concentric hypertrophy is also present. APF = anterior pericardial fluid; PPF = posterior pericardial fluid; IVS = septum; LPW = left ventricular posterior wall; MV = mitral valve; Ao = aorta; LA = left atrium.

heart failure and fluid overload or primary myocardial disease (dilated heart with or without concentric hypertrophy or cardiomyopathic pattern). In all three instances the chest x-ray demonstrated an enlarged heart without being able to differentiate the precise pathophysiologic process. Clinically silent pericardial effusion in patients on long term hemodialysis detected by echocardiography has also been reported by other investigators.[39] These patients should be carefully monitored and observed for the development of cardiac tamponade.

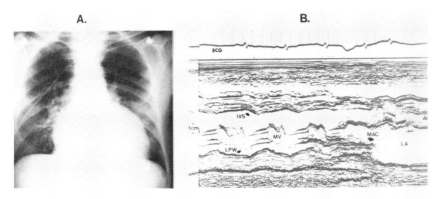

FIGURE 6. A, X-ray in a patient with chronic renal failure and an enlarged heart. B, Same patient demonstrating concentric hypertrophy and mitral annular calcification (MAC). IVS = septum; LPW = left ventricular posterior wall; MV = mitral valve; Ao = aorta; LA = left atrium.

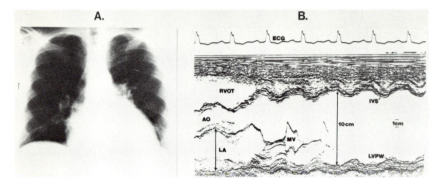

FIGURE 7. A, X-ray in a patient with chronic renal failure and an enlarged heart. B, Same patient demonstrating grossly enlarged left ventricular cavity with diffuse hypokinesia of left ventricular posterior wall (LVPW) and to a lesser extent of the septum (IVS). RVOT = right ventricular outflow tract; Ao = aorta; LA = left atrium.

COMPLICATIONS

Cardiac Tamponade

The most significant complication of uremic pericarditis is cardiac tamponade. It is likely to occur more during or immediately after hemodialysis.[4] In one study reported by Silverberg and associates,[4] cardiac tamponade developed in 15 percent of patients with uremic pericarditis, none of whom was undergoing peritoneal dialysis. It may be extremely difficult to differentiate cardiac tamponade from hypovolemia and increasing heart failure from fluid overload or primary myocardial disease.

In order to determine the hemodynamic effects of a pericardial effusion, cardiac catheterization may be necessary. In severe cases, pulsus paradoxus is recorded from the systemic artery (see Fig. 1). During inspiration, peak arterial systolic pressure declines 15 to 20 mm Hg. The venous and right atrial pressures are elevated often to 20 mm Hg or more. The venous pressure exhibits a normal inspiratory decline and the "y" descent is absent in right atrial pressure tracings, two features that are helpful in differentiating tamponade from constrictive pericarditis. The normal biphasic pattern of venous return is replaced by a monophasic pattern in which venous return is limited to ventricular systole.[23] In addition, inspiration is associated with an increase in venous return and Kussmaul's sign is absent in cardiac tamponade.[24] The ventricular diastolic pressures are elevated and equal to each other and are also equal to the intrapericardial pressure (Fig. 8) in patients without left ven-

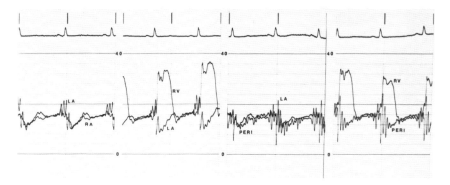

FIGURE 8. Simultaneous·pressure recordings in a patient with chronic renal failure and tamponade. Pressure recordings were recorded in left atrium (LA), right atrium (RA), right ventricle (RV), and pericardium (PERI). Catheter was inserted into pericardium prior to aspiration. Note all diastolic pressures were elevated at 16 mm Hg but equal including LA and RA, RV and LA, LA and PERI, and RV and pericardium.

tricular dysfunction. Following pericardial aspiration, an increase in blood pressure occurs (Fig. 9) and pulsus paradoxus disappears.

Reddy and coworkers[25] have reported on the hemodynamic studies of patients with pericardial effusions and have observed important differences between patients with pericardial effusions but no cardiac tamponade, patients with uncomplicated cardiac tamponade, and those with cardiac tamponade complicating severe left ventricular dysfunction. They have shown that when left ventricular diastolic pressure is severely elevated, equalization of left and right ventricular diastolic pressure, usually a characteristic sign of cardiac tamponade, no longer occurs.[25] In addition, pulsus paradoxus may not be present.[25] The significance of Reddy's observations with regard to chronic renal failure patients is most important. Many patients with chronic renal disease and pericardial effusions on dialysis have left ventricular dysfunction secondary to underlying myocardial involvement, due to associated coronary artery disease or cardiomyopathy. Therefore, patients with chronic renal failure on dialysis with associated moderate to large pericardial effusion and who are deteriorating clinically should be considered for pericardial drainage despite the characteristic absence of hemodynamic findings of cardiac tamponade.

Congestive Heart Failure

Heart failure may complicate the course of uremic pericarditis as a manifestation of primary myocardial disease or as a result of myocar-

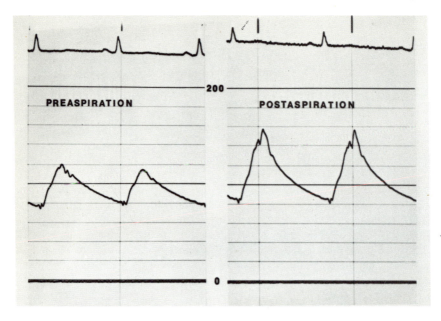

FIGURE 9. Arterial pulse tracings in same patient as in Figure 8. Note the marked increase in arterial pressure postaspiration as compared to preaspiration. BP rose from 120/80 to 158/80.

ditis. A cardiomyopathy has been described by some investigators in patients with end-stage uremia maintained for prolonged periods of time on a low protein diet.[18,19] Massive cardiomegaly, gallop rhythm, hypotension, cardiac arrhythmias, and sensitivity to cardiac glycosides are the characteristic clinical findings. Acute left ventricular failure may occasionally occur in the patient with uremic pericarditis after relief of the pericardial effusion by medical or surgical measures. The clinical syndrome has been reported by Spodick[40] in nonuremic patients and more recently in a patient with severe aortic stenosis and a large pericardial effusion.[41]

Subacute and Chronic Constrictive Pericarditis

Subacute uremic constrictive pericarditis may follow an acute episode immediately or may develop weeks or months later. Hypotension during dialysis may be a prominent clinical manifestation and should alert the physician to this possibility. Symptoms include weight gain, fatigue, dyspnea, and increase in abdominal girth with findings of venous distension, ascites, edema, and hepatomegaly. A friction rub may or may not be audible. The heart, on chest x-ray, may show a decrease in size, and lung fields show no pulmonary vascular congestion.

Chronic constrictive pericarditis appears to be more frequently described in patients who have developed pericarditis on chronic hemodialysis, although it is still a rare complication of uremic pericarditis.[2,42,43] Patients have survived for longer periods of time on chronic hemodialysis. It is clinically indistinguishable from subacute constrictive pericarditis and severe congestive heart failure. Pulsus paradoxus and a pericardial knock may be found in 25 to 65 percent of cases respectively.[44] The pericardial knock is an early diastolic sound occurring approximately 0.09 to 0.12 sec after the aortic component of the second sound and may be mistaken for a third heart sound or an opening snap. Kussmaul's sign (paradoxical distension of the neck veins during inspiration) may occur in constrictive pericarditis.

The value of echocardiography in the diagnosis of constrictive pericarditis is controversial.[45-48] No consistent echocardiographic patterns of pericardial thickening diagnostic of constriction have yet been reported.[48] Seven echocardiographic patterns consistent with pericardial adhesions or pericardial thickening have been recently described by Schnittger and coworkers.[48] The distinction between pericardial thickening patterns and small to moderate pericardial effusions is extremely difficult. Other echocardiographic findings include abnormal septal motion,[45] and a characteristic late diastolic anterior displacement of the septum has been reported.[46] Other suggestive features include flat posterior left ventricular wall motion during diastole and a rapid EF slope.[48]

Cardiac catheterization is essential in patients with suspected constrictive pericarditis. The right atrial pressure does not decline during inspiration and may actually increase (Kussmaul's sign). The "a" and "v" waves are usually of equal amplitude with rapid "x" and "y" descents. The characteristic "M" or "W" form in the venous or right atrial pressure is recorded.[24]

The right ventricular pressure displays a deep early diastolic dip corresponding with and equal to the "y" descent of the right atrial pressure, followed by a rise in pressure and a characteristic plateau configuration.[24] The wave form and amplitude of left ventricular diastolic pressure is almost identical to that of the right ventricle. Pulmonary arterial diastolic pressure is equal to the end-diastolic pressure in the ventricles.[24] The pulmonary wedge pressure is equal to the left ventricular diastolic pressure and has a wave form that closely resembles that of the right atrial pressure.[24] Thus, catheterization usually allows differentiation of constrictive pericarditis from pericardial effusion[24] and cardiomyopathy.[44]

PROGNOSIS

The mortality from uremic pericarditis in the dialyzed patient has been reported to vary between 8 and 20 percent.[7] In a most recent study a high mortality rate of 56 percent was reported.[4] In that study only one patient died because of cardiac tamponade and another of cardiomyopathy.[4] Other causes of death were due to infection, metabolic imbalance, and other cardiovascular lesions.[4] Twenty-one percent of patients die within 2 months of the pericarditis, reflecting the tendency for pericarditis to develop in severely ill patients.[4] The high mortality rate in recent years (1971-1975) has not shown a decline from the years 1966-1970.[7]

TREATMENT

Management of uremic pericarditis is presented in Figure 10. Preventing infection or dehydration coupled with protein restriction may result in improvement in patients with uremic pericarditis who are not in end-

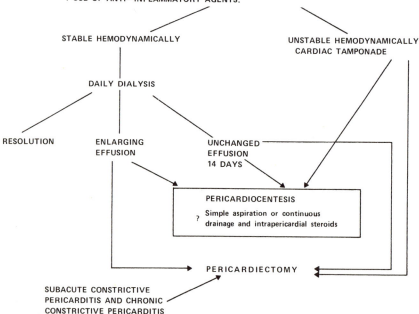

FIGURE 10. Management of uremic pericarditis.

stage renal failure. In these patients appropriate dietary protein restriction, treatment of the acute insult and, occasionally, a single peritoneal dialysis will result in clinical resolution of pericarditis.[7]

Several studies have shown that up to one-half or more of the patients with hemodynamically stable uremic effusions are managed safely by intensive dialysis.[2,5,7] In patients who have already been treated with chronic hemodialysis and the effusion has not dramatically resolved, inadequate dialysis may have resulted from a malfunctioning access or because of missed dialysis.[3] Measurements of peroneal nerve conduction velocity should be undertaken because if there has been progression of uremic neuropathy it would suggest inadequate dialysis.[7] Most centers increase dialysis therapy by at least 30 percent over the previous dialysis with regard to duration and/or frequency in patients with the diagnosis of uremic pericarditis.[7] During the process of increased dialysis, careful attention should be paid to nutrition.[7] With increased dialysis, losses of essential amino acids may occur resulting in a catabolic state.[7] Adequate calories plus supplementary amino acid mixtures are essential.

Anticoagulants should be discontinued until active pericarditis has resolved. The harmful effects of heparin can be avoided by using regional heparinization[7] or by employing peritoneal dialysis.[49] Peritoneal dialysis may be the treatment of choice for the initiation of dialysis therapy in patients with uremic pericarditis since it avoids the danger of heparinization in a patient with hemorrhagic tendency and acutely inflamed serous membranes.[7]

It may be difficult to balance fluid requirements in the patient with uremic pericarditis. Overhydration and heart failure have to be carefully balanced between maintenance of adequate blood volume in a patient with a large pericardial effusion and compression. In addition, sudden changes in intravascular volume during dialysis must be avoided. Where it is extremely difficult to differentiate between hypovolemia and shock or cardiac tamponade, or fluid overload and congestive heart failure, a Swan-Ganz catheter should be inserted to determine right heart and wedge pressures. If severe congestive heart failure is present with fluid overload, some degree of fluid removal by ultrafiltration becomes essential.[7] Digitalis in the management of uremic pericarditis is controversial. In the presence of supraventricular tachycardias, digitalis should be used, but its use in renal failure requires modification and careful attention should be paid to potassium levels.

The use of anti-inflammatory drugs remains controversial. Indomethacin, an antipyretic and anti-inflammatory agent, has been used without dosage modification in renal failure with success in the treatment of uremic pericarditis.[50] Pain abated within 6 to 24 hours in most patients. When treatment was discontinued during the first week, symptoms recurred. In most instances, the drug could be tapered and discontinued after 3 weeks to 4 months. Other investigators have reported a beneficial effect with the use of prednisone (40 mg daily).[2,42] A dramatic disappearance of pain, subsidence of fever, diminution of friction rub, and reduction of the heart size have been reported.[2,42] If the patient responds to steroids during the first week of therapy, steroids should be gradually tapered and withdrawn by the end of 4 to 6 weeks. However, oral steroid administration, although frequently successful, may be complicated by the necessity for prolonged administration and frequent complications such as sepsis, gastrointestinal hemorrhage, and the recurrence of pericarditis after cessation.

The role of pericardiocentesis in the therapy of uremic pericardial effusion and tamponade is also controversial.[7] Reported complications of pericardiocentesis include the development of acute tamponade without evidence of myocardial injury, coronary artery lacerations, and ventricular perforations.[51-53] Bloody pericardial fluid is commonly found in patients on long term dialysis and because of the coagulopathy of uremia, repeated attempts at pericardiocentesis may be associated with bleeding and accelerated cardiac tamponade. A mortality as high as 75 percent has been reported with pericardiocentesis in patients with uremic pericarditis.[52] There have been several reports stressing the effectiveness of catheter drainage and intrapericardial steroids in the treatment of patients with "intractable" uremic pericardial effusions.[54-58] The technique of pericardial triamcinolone hexacetonide instillation was first described by Buselmeier and coworkers.[54] After instillation of local anesthesia and intramuscular atropine, a 16 gauge, 13.3 cm steel needle with a plastic outer sheath is inserted subxiphoid and directed toward the left shoulder. The needle is connected to chest lead of an electrocardiograph to monitor injury currents. When resistance is noted, the stylet is removed and a guidance is then inserted through the cannula under fluoroscopic control. With the guide wire in place, the cannula is then removed. A polyethylene catheter is then advanced over the guide wire for a length of 15.3 cm and the guide wire is then removed. After removal of pericardial fluid, 50 mg of triamcinolone hexacetonide is instilled into the pericardial sac. The removal of fluid and instillation of steroids and heparin sodium are repeated every 4 to 6 hours until less than 10 ml of pericardial fluid is obtained. Frequent cultures of the aspirated fluid are obtained to detect bacterial contamination. Fuller and colleagues[55] employing this technique treated 5 patients with intractable pericarditis unresponsive to intensive dialysis and pericardiocentesis. Pericardial drainage was prolonged and ranged from 19 to 60 hours. The average total dose of steroid instilled was 370 mg with a range of 200 to 500 mg and signs and symptoms abated on an average of 3 days (range of 1 to 7 days). All 5 patients recovered and were subsequently observed from 1 to 15 months with no evidence of recurrent pericarditis. Buselmeier and coworkers[56] updated their experience by reporting on the effectiveness of catheter drainage and intrapericardial steroids in the treatment of 24 patients with "intractable" uremic pericardial effusions. Oakes and others[57] reported on the successful effect of pericardiocentesis and single-dose instillation of triamcinolone hexacetonide.

A variety of surgical approaches combined with local or extensive pericardiectomy has been recommended.[51-53,59] Most series have reported low mortality and morbidity rates.[51-53,59] Usually, constrictive pericarditis has been prevented following pericardiectomy. Connors and associates[59] reported on 16 patients who underwent a left anterior thoractomy with extensive anterior pericardiectomy and the creation of a small window posterior to the phrenic nerve. Their indications for surgery included cardiac tamponade, enlarging effusions or those unchanged in size while on dialysis, and hypotension on dialysis.[59] Additional indications for pericardiectomy include patients with subacute constrictive pericarditis who have developed hypotension, hepatomegaly, ascites and edema,[32] as well as patients with chronic constrictive pericarditis and severe right heart failure.[7] No operative deaths were reported but significant morbidity occurred in three patients. After an average followup period of 33.9 months following operation, subacute or chronic constrictive pericarditis had not developed.[59] Median sternotomy with wide resection of the anterior pericardium appears to be an unwarranted and unnecessary procedure in uremic pericardial effusion.[59] The subxiphoid approach under local anesthesia should be avoided because it does not consistently provide adequate exposure for complete adhesiolysis.[59]

SUMMARY

The incidence of uremic pericarditis occurs in 14 to 20 percent of patients undergoing dialysis. No single etiologic factor can be implicated as a cause of uremic pericarditis. Chest pain, fever, and a pericardial friction rub are the three most common clinical manifestations. The electrocardiogram is of minimal value in the diagnosis of uremic pericarditis. Echocardiography is the simplest, safest, and probably the most accurate method of diagnosing pericardial fluid. The most significant complication of uremic pericarditis is cardiac tamponade. It occurs in 15 percent of patients with uremic pericarditis. Cardiac tamponade is a clinical diagnosis. It may be recognized by the development of hypotension during the course of hemodialysis coupled with neck vein engorgement, tachycardia, and pulsus paradoxus. However, in the presence of severe hypotension or in severe left ventricular failure, pulsus paradoxus may *not* be recognized. Under such circumstances cardiac catheterization may be necessary to determine the hemodynamics of a pericardial effusion.

Additional complications include congestive heart failure due to left ventricular dysfunction and/or fluid overload. Subacute and chronic constrictive pericarditis may rarely follow an acute episode immediately, but may occur weeks or months later. Although echocardiography may be helpful in the differential diagnosis of the spectrum of cardiac involvement in chronic renal failure, cardiac catheterization may be necessary to define the precise pathophysiologic disorder.

The management of uremic pericarditis is controversial. While there is general agreement with regard to biochemical control, nutrition, fluid balance, treatment of arrhythmias, and increased need for dialysis, there has been disagreement with regard to the use of anti-inflammatory agents, pericardiocentesis, and pericardiectomy. In the presence of tamponade, pericardial drainage is mandatory and if simple aspiration is unsuccessful pericardiectomy and drainage may be necessary. Pericardial drainage should be considered in patients whose effusion has not changed over a 14 day period or appears to be enlarging despite an adequate dialysis program. In patients who are clinically symptomatic with subacute or chronic constrictive pericarditis, pericardiectomy should be performed.

REFERENCES

1. Bright, R.: Tubular view of the morbid appearance in 100 cases connected with albuminous urine: with observations. Guys Hosp. Rep. 1:338, 1836.
2. Comty, C.M., Cohen, S.L., and Shapiro, F.L.: Pericarditis in chronic uremia and its sequels. Ann. Intern. Med. 75:173, 1971.
3. Ribot, S., Frankel, H.J., Gielchinsky, I., et al.: Treatment of uremic pericarditis. Clin. Nephrol. 2:127, 1974.
4. Silverberg, S., Oreopoulos, D.G., Wise, D.J., et al.: Pericarditis in patients undergoing long-term hemodialysis and peritoneal dialysis. Incidence, complications and management. Am. J. Med. 63:874, 1977.
5. Bailey, G.L., Hampers, C.L., Hager, E.B., et al.: Uremic pericarditis: clinical features and management. Circulation 38:582, 1968.
6. Wacker, W., and Merrill, J.P.: Uremic pericarditis in acute and chronic renal failure. JAMA 156:764, 1954.
7. Comty, C.M., Wathen, R.L., and Shapiro, F.L.: Uremic pericarditis, *in* Spodick, D.H. (ed.): Pericardial Diseases. F.A. Davis, Philadelphia, 1976, p. 219.
8. Holt, J.P.: The normal pericardium. Am. J. Cardiol. 26:455, 1970.
9. Miller, A.J., Pick, R., and Johnson, P.J.: Lymphatic drainage of the heart. Am. J. Cardiol. 26:463, 1971.
10. Avasthey, P., and Wood, E.H.: Intrathoracic and venous pressure relation-

ships during responses to changes in body position. J. Appl. Physiol. 37:166, 1974.

11. Spotnitz, H.M., and Kaiser, G.A.: The effect of the pericardium on pressure-volume relations in the canine left ventricle. J. Surg. Res. 11:375, 1971.

12. Hefner, L.L., Coghlan, H.C., Jones, W.B., et al.: Distensibility of the dog left ventricle. Am. J. Physiol. 201:97, 1962.

13. Shirato, K., Shabetai, R., Bhargova, V., et al.: Alteration of the left ventricular diastolic pressure-segment length relation produced by the pericardium. Effects of cardiac distention and afterload reduction in conscious dogs. Circulation 57:1191, 1977.

14. Beaudry, G., Nakamoto, S., and Kolff, W.J.: Uremic pericarditis and tamponade in chronic renal failure. Ann. Intern. Med. 64:990, 1966.

15. Luft, F.C., Kleit, S.A., Smith, R.N., et al.: Management of uremic pericarditis with tamponade. Arch. Intern. Med. 134:488, 1974.

16. Skov, S.E., Hansen, H.E., and Spencer, E.S.: Uremic pericarditis. Acta Med. Scand. 186:421, 1969.

17. Pabico, R.C., Hanshaw, J.B., and Talley, T.E.: Cytomegalovirus infection in chronic hemodialysis patients. Abstr. West. Dialysis and Transplantation Soc., Oct. 9–10, 1971.

18. Bailey, G.L., Hampers, C.L., and Merrill, J.P.: Reversible cardiomyopathy in uremia. Trans. Am. Soc. Artif. Intern. Organs 13:263, 1967.

19. Lanhez, L.E., Lowen, J., and Sabbaga, E.: Uremic myocardiopathy. Nephrol. 15:17, 1975.

20. Dunn, M., and Rinkenberger, R.L.: Clinical aspects of acute pericarditis, in Spodick, D.H. (ed.): Pericardial Diseases. F.A. Davis Company, Philadelphia, 1976, p. 131.

21. Spodick, D.H.: Pericardial rub; prospective, multiple observer investigation of pericardial friction in 100 patients. Am. J. Cardiol. 35:357, 1975.

22. Kuhn, L.A.: Acute and chronic cardiac tamponade, in Spodick, D.H. (ed.): Pericardial Diseases. F.A. Davis Company, Philadelphia, 1976, p. 177.

23. Shabetai, R., Fowler, N.O., and Guntheroth, W.G.: The hemodynamics of cardiac tamponade and constrictive pericarditis. Am. J. Cardiol. 26:480, 1970.

24. Shabetai, R.: The pathophysiology of cardiac tamponade and constriction, in Spodick, D.H. (ed.): Pericardial Diseases. F.A. Davis Company, Philadelphia, 1976, p. 67.

25. Reddy, P.S., Curtiss, E.I., O'Toole, J.E., et al.: Cardiac tamponade: hemodynamic observations in man. Circulation 58:265, 1978.

26. Horowitz, M.S., Schultz, C.S., Stinson, E.B., et al.: Sensitivity and specificity of echocardiographic diagnosis of pericardial effusion. Circulation 50:239, 1974.

27. Tajik, A.J.: Echocardiography in pericardial effusion. Am. J. Med. 63:29, 1977.

28. Lemire, F., Tajik, A.J., Giulani, E.R., et al.: Further echocardiographic observations in pericardial effusion. Mayo Clin. Proc. 51:13, 1976.

29. Nanda, N.C., Gramiak, R., and Gross, C.M.: Echocardiography of cardiac valves in pericardial effusion. Circulation 54:500, 1976.

30. Owens, J.S., Kotler, M.N., Segal, B.L., et al.: Pseudoprolapse of the mitral valve in a patient with pericardial effusion. Chest 69:214, 1976.

31. Gabor, G.E., Winsberg, F., and Bloom, H.S.: Electrical and mechanical alteration in pericardial effusion. Chest 59:341, 1971.

32. Usher, B.W., and Popp, R.L.: Electrical alternans, mechanism in pericardial effusion. Am. Heart J. 83:459, 1972.
33. Kotler, M.N., Segal, B.L., Mintz, G., et al.: Pitfalls and limitations of M-mode echocardiography. Am. Heart J. 94:227, 1977.
34. Schott, C.R., Kotler, M.N., Parry, W.R., et al.: Mitral annular calcification. Clinical and echocardiographic correlations. Arch. Intern. Med. 137:1143, 1977.
35. D'Cruz, I.A., Cohen, H.C., Prabhu, R., et al.: Diagnosis of cardiac tamponade by echocardiography. Changes in mitral valve motion and ventricular dimensions, with special reference to paradoxic pulse. Circulation 52:460, 1975.
36. Vignola, P.A., Pohost, G.M., Curfman, G.E., et al.: Correlation of echocardiographic and clinical findings in patients with pericardial effusion. Am. J. Cardiol. 37:701, 1976.
37. Schiller, N.B., and Botvinick, E.H.: Right ventricular compression as a sign of cardiac tamponade. An analysis of echocardiographic ventricular dimensions and their clinical implications. Circulation 56:774, 1977.
38. Schott, C.R., LeSar, J.F., Kotler, M.N., et al.: The spectrum of echocardiographic findings in chronic renal failure. Cardiovasc. Med. 3:217, 1978.
39. Goldstein, D.H., Nagar, C., Srivastava, N., et al.: Clinically silent pericardial effusions in patients on long-term hemodialysis. Pericardial effusions in hemodialysis. Chest 72:744, 1977.
40. Spodick, D.H.: Acute cardiac tamponade: pathologic physiology, diagnosis and management. Prog. Cardiovasc. Dis. 10:64, 1967.
41. Wheatley, C.E.: Acute idiopathic pericarditis and calcific aortic stenosis: unusual fatal disease combination. Am. Heart J. 96:87, 1978.
42. Wolfe, S.A., Bailey, G.F., and Collins, J.J., Jr.: Constrictive pericarditis following uremic effusion. J. Thorac. Cardiovasc. Surg. 63:540, 1972.
43. Lindsay, J., Jr., Crawley, I.S., and Callaway, G.M.: Chronic constrictive pericarditis following uremic hemopericardium. Am. Heart J. 79:390, 1970.
44. Wise, D.E., and Conti, C.R.: Constrictive pericarditis, in Spodick, D.H. (ed.): Pericardial Diseases. F.A. Davis Company, Philadelphia, 1976, p. 197.
45. Pool, P.E., Seagren, S.C., Abbasi, A.S., et al.: Echocardiographic manifestations of constrictive pericarditis—abnormal septal motion. Chest 68:684, 1975.
46. Gibson, T.C., Grossman, W., and McLaurin, L.P.: An echocardiographic study of the interventricular septum in constrictive pericarditis. Br. Heart J. 38:738, 1976.
47. Elkayam, U., Kotler, M.N., Segal, B.L., et al.: Echocardiographic findings in constrictive pericarditis. Israel J. Med. Sci. 12:1308, 1976.
48. Schnittger, I., Bowden, R.E., Abrams, J., et al.: Echocardiography: pericardial thickening and constrictive pericarditis. Am. J. Cardiol. 42:388, 1978.
49. Cohen, G.F., Burgess, J.H., and Kaye, M.: Peritoneal dialysis for the treatment of pericarditis in patients on chronic hemodialysis. Canad. Med. Assoc. J. 102:1365, 1970.
50. Minuth, A.N.W., Nottebohn, G.A., Eknoyan, G., et al.: Indomethacin treatment of pericarditis in chronic hemodialysis patients. Arch. Intern. Med. 135:807, 1975.
51. Ghavamian, M., Gutch, C.F., Hughes, R.K., et al.: Pericardial tamponade in chronic hemodialysis patients. Treatment by pericardiectomy. Arch. Intern. Med. 131:249, 1973.

52. Singh, Newmark K., and Ishikawa, I., et al.: Pericardiectomy in uremia. JAMA 228:1132, 1974.
53. Wray, T.M., Humphreys, J., Perry, J.M., et al.: Pericardiectomy for treatment of uremic pericarditis. Circulation 50 (Suppl. II):268, 1974.
54. Buselmeier, T.J., Simmons, R.G., Najarian, J.S., et al.: Intractable uremic pericardial effusion. Proc. Eur. Dialy. Transpl. For. 55:1973.
55. Fuller, T.J., Knockel, J.P., Brennan, J.P., et al.: Reversal of intractable uremic pericarditis by triamcinolone hexacetonide. Arch. Intern. Med. 136:979, 1976.
56. Buselmeier, T.J., Simmons, R.L., Mauer, S.M., et al.: Pericardiectomy. Surgery 82:170, 1972.
57. Oakes, D.D., Weidig, J.C., and Spees, E.K.: Another view on treatment for uremic pericardial effusion. Surgery 82:894, 1977.
58. Spodick, D.H.: The management of uremic pericardial effusion. Surgery 83:609, 1978.
59. Connors, J.P., Klieger, R.E., and Shaw, R.C.: The indications for pericardiectomy in the uremic pericardial effusion. Surgery 80:689, 1976.
60. Cochran, M., Lawton, S., and Rowlands, L.N.: Fibrinous pericarditis and fibrinolysis in chronic dialysis patients. Clin. Nephrol. 11:23, 1979.
61. Cohen, M.V., Diaz, P., and Scheuer, J.: Echocardiographic assessment of left ventricular function in patients with chronic uremia. Clin. Nephrol. 12:156, 1979.

6

ATHEROSCLEROSIS AND ITS COMPLICATIONS

STUART SNYDER, M.D., WILLIAM LIKOFF, M.D., AND RONALD PENNOCK, M.D.,

PATHOGENESIS

While the exact mechanism(s) for the increased rate of atherosclerosis[1-3] and its complications in chronic renal failure has not yet been ascertained and has in fact been vigorously challenged,[4,5] there are a number of known abnormalities that may be present in patients with chronic renal failure and may be responsible for the increased risk of atherosclerosis. In the first place, it is well known that plasma high density lipoprotein levels are inversely related to the incidence of atherosclerosis in various population groups.[6] High density lipoprotein appears to have some protective value against the development of coronary heart disease. Furthermore, in circumstances in which patients have protection from atherosclerosis, that is, in females and youth, levels of high density lipoprotein appear to be increased. On the other hand, in states that appear to produce a predisposition to atherosclerosis, such as obesity, diabetes, or hypertension, the levels of high density lipoproteins are conversely decreased. In addition, smokers also have a decreased level of high density lipoproteins.[7] The mechanism for the effect of high density lipoprotein is not entirely ascertained, but there is evidence that the high density lipoprotein molecule may facilitate the transport of cholesterol from the arterial wall, or may even affect the uptake of low density lipoprotein by the arterial wall. Studies of this lipoprotein in renal disease have shown that high density lipoprotein levels are significantly reduced either in patients undergoing hemodialysis or in patients who have undergone renal transplantation when compared to controls.[8] The

111

mechanism for this reduction is not known at this point, but the decrease in high density lipoproteins could certainly be part of the explanation for the acceleration of atherogenesis in chronic renal disease. Furthermore, many patients with chronic renal failure are hypertensive and this may likewise be a partial mechanism in their increased risk of atherogenesis.

In addition, there appears to be a relationship between levels of immunoreactive growth hormone and blood sugar, to blood lipids, and perhaps even to atherosclerosis. Moreover, recent studies have shown that immunoreactive growth hormone levels in patients with chronic renal failure seem to be elevated.[9] These changes, likewise, may have some relationship to the increased risk of atherosclerosis in chronic renal failure.

However, of all the abnormalities which might be related to atherosclerosis, the one which has been most extensively studied is hyperlipidemia. Hyperlipidemia does appear to be frequent in postrenal transplant patients and those undergoing chronic hemodialysis. In one study,[10] 61 percent of postrenal transplant patients had hyperlipidemia. In this particular study, levels of both serum cholesterol and triglycerides were significantly elevated and many of the patients had a type II disorder. In contrast, most other studies have shown that the predominant disorder in patients on hemodialysis or postrenal transplant appears to be hypertriglyceridemia rather than hypercholesterolemia.[11,12]

While the exact etiology for the development of hypertriglyceridemia certainly is not entirely clear, in some patients it seems to be related to increased serum insulin levels.[12] In contrast, hypertriglyceridemia does not appear to be related to obesity in these patients. Moreover, the insulin resistance noted in chronic renal failure appears to produce increased hepatic triglyceride synthesis by itself, and any increased dietary carbohydrate content in these patients does not appear to be a significant factor in hepatic synthesis. In addition, there also appears to be a defect in triglyceride removal in chronic renal disease which apparently is a result of decreased activity of tissue lipoprotein lipase.[12] In contrast, other studies have shown a concomitant selective decrease of hepatic triglyceride lipase with a normal lipoprotein lipase activity.[13] Other authors have actually identified a circulating plasma protein which inhibits lipoprotein lipase.[14] Regardless of the mechanism involved, however, there is well documented hyperglyceridemia in patients with chronic uremia or after renal transplant, and this may be related to the acceleration of atherogenesis in addition to other known factors which also could accelerate atherogenesis in this condition.

Most patients who have hypertriglyceridemia in the absence of renal failure can be shown to have one or more underlying etiologies, for example, hypothyroidism, diabetes mellitus, and alcoholism. In addition to

a hereditary predisposition, the diet of these patients may consist of excessive carbohydrate and simple sugar intake; they may drink considerable quantities of alcohol, may be obese, and may have glucose intolerance. Other patients may have been taking steroids or estrogens.
However, in the case of patients with chronic renal failure and hypertriglyceridemia, the interaction of these usual risk factors for the development of hypertriglyceridemia may not be apparent. If the patient is
receiving steroids or is on a very high carbohydrate, low protein diet,
then these usual factors could be partially causal. However, hypertriglyceridemia does appear to occur in patients with chronic renal failure
without necessarily having any of the usual predisposing factors for this
beyond their chronic renal failure itself.

MANAGEMENT

The usual treatment for hypertriglyceridemia in patients without chronic
renal failure would be weight loss, control of glucose intolerance,
decrease in the intake of carbohydrates and simple sugars, and a reduction of alcohol ingestion. In many patients adherence to a diet and
significant reduction of weight will result in a marked decrease in the
triglyceride levels. However, in the case of patients with chronic renal
disease and hypertriglyceridemia, there is no evidence that correction of
the usual predisposing factors causes any reduction in triglyceride levels.
In addition, some patients are given androgens (for the normochromic
normocytic anemia of chronic renal failure), which may worsen the
hypertriglyceridemia.[15] Therefore, if it is possible to reduce the dosage of
steroids or androgens, then this could possibly result in lipid lowering.
   Drug therapy for the treatment of hypertriglyceridemia in nonuremic
patients has been highly controversial.[16] For several years, clofibrate was
recommended for certain types of hypertriglyceridemia. However, a review of the results of the Coronary Drug Project[17] has indicated no
change in mortality but a significant increase in morbidity in terms of angina, claudication, and gallstones[17] in patients who received clofibrate.
This study was done, however, using patients who had already suffered a
myocardial infarction and did not evaluate any other type of patients, for
example, those with uremia or diabetes or patients with hyperlipidemia.
In contradistinction to those studies, there are data to suggest that clofibrate can increase lipoprotein lipase and high density lipoprotein cholesterol in patients on dialysis[18-20] and after renal transplantation. Elevated
blood levels of clofibrate are seen in chronic renal failure.[21] The plasma
protein binding is impaired giving rise to an increase in free clofibrate for
pharmacologic activity and possible toxicity.[22,23]
   Other drugs which have been used to treat hypertriglyceridemia, such

as nicotinic acid and thyroxine, have not been studied in patients with uremia. In a review of the Coronary Drug Project,[17] d-thyroxine was shown to be associated with an increased mortality for patients with past myocardial infarction. Similarly, nicotinic acid did not significantly affect morbidity in these patients. These drugs might be used for the treatment of hypertriglyceridemia but their usefulness in patients with known coronary artery disease is questionable. Therefore, with the highly controversial nature of lipid lowering agents in patients in hypertriglyceridemia, they could not be recommended except in the most unusual circumstances for patients having chronic renal failure and hyperlipidemia.

SUMMARY

It appears that a very common disorder of patients undergoing chronic dialysis or after renal transplantation is hyperlipidemia, and the most common variety of this hyperlipidemia is hypertriglyceridemia. Studies suggest that clofibrate may be efficacious. In addition, these patients may have continuing factors that would tend to propagate the hypertriglyceridemia, such as the requirements for steroids, high carbohydrate diet, continued glucose intolerance, or the acetate content of the dialysis bath, a known precursor of free fatty acid and glycerol synthesis.[24]

Unfortunately, in spite of optimum control of lipogenic factors, ischemic heart disease can develop and the anginal syndrome may be the first clue to its existence.

ANGINA SYNDROME OF CORONARY ARTERY DISEASE

Angina pectoris is essentially a manifestation of myocardial ischemia that results from an imbalance between available oxygen supply and the demands of the myocardium. The former depends upon coronary flow which, in turn, is mainly regulated by the internal caliber of the coronary arteries. Atherosclerosis is the most common cause of a reduction in the caliber of these vessels, usually being widely distributed and seriously obstructive in the majority of patients with the anginal syndrome.

Angina also occurs when the coronary arteries are normally patent. In these instances, a mechanism other than organic obstruction accounts for upsetting the balance between coronary flow and the nutritional needs of the myocardium. For example, in aortic stenosis the marked elevation of intraventricular pressure increases peripheral coronary resistance, thereby diminishing coronary blood flow during systole. At the same time, myocardial metabolic needs are increased because of the thickened left ventricular musculature, the high intraventricular pressure, and the prolonged ejection interval.

Subjects with aortic regurgitation may suffer from angina pectoris in spite of an overdeveloped and widely patent coronary arterial circulation. Factors held responsible include diminished coronary blood flow brought on by abnormally low aortic diastolic pressure and the size and configuration of the dilated left ventricle resulting in increased myocardial oxygen consumption.

Mechanisms responsible for angina in restrictive and congestive cardiomyopathies are less certain but may include metabolic errors impeding oxygen utilization at a cellular level. In these instances, as well as angina at rest, the concept of coronary arterial spasm also has been invoked as an explanation for myocardial ischemia.

Knowledge pertaining to the pathophysiology of angina pectoris, however incomplete, is by far more advanced than representations regarding the origin of atherosclerosis which, as has been stated previously, is the most common source of obstructive coronary disease. Although the specific cause of atherosclerosis is unknown, a number of factors are believed to favor its development. Among the more significant are hypertension (see Chapters 2 and 9) and hyperlipidemia.

Accordingly, it follows that patients with chronic renal failure undergoing maintenance hemodialysis are *believed* to have both a greater incidence of atherosclerotic cardiovascular disease and an uncommonly accelerated evolutionary pattern of such ailments. Indeed, it is reported that approximately 30 percent of chronic dialysis patient deaths are due to cardiovascular causes.[2] More than one-third of these deaths are due to myocardial infarction. However, long term followup studies of ischemic heart disease (IHD) in patients undergoing maintenance hemodialysis show that the rate of IHD in female dialysis patients was greater than in nondialysis subjects, that coronary artery disease affected survival in patients with pre-existing disease, and that postmortem data showed no accelerated atherosclerosis.[4]

Diagnosis

The diagnosis of angina pectoris in an individual with chronic renal failure is essentially based upon the report of a transient, but insistent and compelling discomfort in the midchest, or in the epigastrium. Classically, this occurs with effort and progresses to a peak in the course of which it may radiate into the neck, jaws, teeth, hands, and most frequently the left arm.

The sensation—as Heberden so aptly stated approximately 200 years ago—may be associated with a feeling that life itself is about to be extinguished. Then, with time and rest, it gradually subsides, leaving the patient with either no apparent disability or in a somewhat exhausted and frightened state.

The quality of the discomfort is variously described as crushing, oppressive, heavy, or burning. Only rarely is it said to be "a pain." Despite these variations in character, the sensation usually is the same from episode to episode in any given patient.

Although the discomfort is usually retrosternal and in the midchest, it may be experienced over the entire precordium as well as in the area between the shoulder blades, and more occasionally in the lower back where it is mistakenly thought to be arthritis or neuromuscular disease.

Patients with angina pectoris often define the location of the chest discomfort by placing a hand across the front portion of the chest, clinching the fist to convey the quality of the sensation. Rarely, if ever, does an individual point to the area with an isolated finger or two.

A number of conditions may be confused with the diagnosis of angina pectoris, including neuromuscular conditions of the chest wall, hiatal hernia, esophagitis, esophageal spasm and reflux, cardiac dysrhythmias, and dissection of the aorta. In the patient with chronic renal failure, acute pericarditis may present with subjective complaints strikingly akin to angina pectoris. The presence of chills, fever, leukocytosis, friction rub, and gallop rhythm materially may assist in making a very difficult differential diagnosis.

The remarkable fact about the physical examination of the heart in patients with angina is that it is so often normal. However, in the presence of chronic renal failure, this is not the rule. Hypertension is a common abnormality. The murmur of aortic insufficiency frequently is heard at the second and third left interspaces.[25] Gallop rhythm is not unusual. Abnormal cardiac rhythm may be a transient or permanent finding.

Whereas the resting electrocardiogram usually is normal in the majority of patients with angina pectoris, it is clearly abnormal in individuals who also have chronic renal failure. The most common of the abnormalities are manifestations of left ventricular hypertrophy, old myocardial infarction, drug effects, and supraventrical arrhythmias.

In those instances where a carefully defined history, thorough physical examination, and resting electrocardiogram cannot establish a correct diagnosis, special investigation may be necessary. Included among the tests are stress electrocardiography alone or in combination with nuclear myocardial imaging and coronary arteriography. However, each of these is much more difficult to apply and interpret in the presence of chronic renal failure than in its absence.

The ability of patients with chronic renal failure to accommodate to the rigors of stress testing generally is limited. All of the exercise tests subject the individual to either a prefixed load determined by age, sex, and weight or a maximal stress that will cause heart rate to rise to the calculated value for a subject of that age, sex, and weight. In either instance, the requirement is a considerable physical obligation for the debilitated renal patient.

The broad spectrum of chronic renal failure embraces individuals in whom angiographic studies, such as coronary visualization, threaten a delicately balanced clinical state. Those who are hypertensive and given to wide swings of circulating volume with each ultrafiltration are particularly vulnerable. In these patients, angiography as well as stress testing should be performed when blood volume and biochemical balance has been restored to the most reasonable values possible.

It is axiomatic that stress testing and coronary arteriography should be performed only when the information they will provide is essential to diagnosis or treatment. Although the mortality rate associated with exercise electrocardiography is inconsequential even in the presence of chronic renal failure, the test is temporarily incapacitating, costly, and time consuming. Coronary visualization, on the other hand, is associated with an overall mortality rate of 0.1 to 5 percent with the greater risks in subjects with chronic renal failure. Furthermore, it is the cause of much anxiety as well as fear and cannot be carried out unless the patient is hospitalized.

The special studies used in the diagnosis of angina pectoris are remarkably accurate.[26] However, the presence and extent of graphic abnormalities cannot always be correlated with the extent of the physical disability. Patients with grossly abnormal electrocardiograms and severely constricted coronary arteries may from time to time enjoy a better clinical course than those who have relatively limited vascular pathology.

Treatment

The physician's first responsibility is to make certain the patient understands his or her disease. Patients who have been informed of the anatomic and physiologic rudiments of ischemic heart disease are usually the most cooperative.

The patient should also understand that many aspects of management are based more on concept than demonstrable fact. This should help to place in proper perspective the many and various claims made regarding the etiology of atherosclerotic heart disease and should serve as a buffer against the hosts of claims about unproved measures such as weight and dietary controls.

It is generally of value to explain that all risk factors should be eliminated. This includes a prudent diet, a regulated exercise program, avoidance of unusual stress—both physical and mental, absolute cessation of cigarette smoking, control of diabetes, and control of hypertension. Instruction regarding physical activity should be specific, including the amount and type of exercise as well as how often and how long practiced. Patients with chronic renal failure undoubtedly will be forced to accept limited exercise obligations and will find it necessary to correlate those efforts with dialysis. Special caution will have to be exercised for hypertensive and anemic subjects, as well as those who respond to dialysis with wide variations in volume. The frequency and severity of angina is greatly augmented when the concentration of hemoglobin or circulating volume falls significantly.

Sublingual nitroglycerin is the primary medication for angina pectoris and should be used promptly at the onset of pain. Chronic renal failure does not modify the indications for the drug or manner in which it should be administered. Relief of discomfort following the use of nitroglycerin is helpful in confirming the diagnosis of angina. Nitroglycerin can also be used prophylactically if the patient can predict what physical or emotional stress will precipitate the attack.

The dose of nitroglycerin varies from grains 1/100 to 1/200. Effective response to a sublingual tablet should be experienced 2 to 5 minutes after using a fresh tablet. Repeated doses within a short interval may produce hypotension and cause vertigo or actual syncope. It is reasonable to expect that an interval of 15 min should pass before judging the effectiveness of a given dose of nitroglycerin.

Patients should carry a fresh preparation of nitroglycerin routinely. It is unlikely that individual tablets of the standard drug remain potent in a simple pill box longer than 3 to 4 months. Special preparations, however, are available which retain potency for much longer periods of time.

Nitroglycerin is also available in ointment form which, when applied to and absorbed from the skin, is effective in preventing or ameliorating the discomfort of angina pectoris. This preparation has a particular use in the treatment of patients with chronic renal failure because of its prophylactic role.

A number of nitrates, taken sublingually or orally, are available for the treatment of angina pectoris. They are said to reduce preload by virtue of venous pooling. The dose of these agents and the time interval of administration are not altered by the presence of chronic renal failure.

Propranolol hydrochloride is one of the most effective drugs used in the treatment of moderate to severe angina pectoris. The major action of propranolol depresses sympathetic tone thereby decreasing heart rate and contractility and reducing myocardial oxygen requirements. Additionally, the drug decreases the rate of rise of ventricular pressure, increases refractory period in AV mode, and increases left ventricular volume.

Clearance of propranolol depends on hepatic blood flow (Chapter 3). Maintenance dose intervals are unchanged in all degrees of renal failure. Blood levels are the best guide to toxic effects. Major side effects include bradycardia, heart failure, bronchospasm, transient gastrointestinal distress, and varying degrees of fatigue. Furthermore, angina may be complicated by heart failure (Chapter 7), arrhythmias (Chapter 8) and hypertension (Chapter 9). The pathogenesis and treatment of these complications are subsequently reviewed.

Clearly, the medical management of angina pectoris in patients with chronic renal failure varies greatly with the individual, depending upon the severity of the coronary insufficiency and the presence or absence of hypertension and heart failure. Regretably, elevated blood pressure and myocardial failure commonly coexist and require multidrug therapy. In such instances, knowledge of the pharmacokinetics of each agent alone and in combination is necessary if a successful program is to be conducted (see Chapter 3). Nevertheless, even with careful management of the anginal syndrome, acute myocardial infarction may ensue.

MANAGEMENT OF ACUTE MYOCARDIAL INFARCTION

Incidence

Most epidemiologic studies indicate that myocardial infarction accounts for at least 10 percent of deaths in chronic renal failure.[27] At age 25 to 45 in the United States, the cardiovascular death rate in chronic renal failure[28,29] is three to four times higher than in similar age patients with normal kidney function. In the National Dialysis Registry Death Analysis of April 1976,[30] over 600 deaths at an average age of 55 were attributed to myocardial infarction. Mahoney and coworkers[31] showed that once a chronic renal failure patient has evidence of coronary artery disease, subsequent renal transplantation did not prevent myocardial infarction from occurring. The statement is made that patients should be considered for transplantation only if they have neither angina nor previous myocardial infarction.

In the 12th Report of the Human Renal Transplant Registry,[32] 193 recipients of transplants died of myocardial infarction at an average age of 41 years. According to their statistics, nephrosclerosis and diabetes mellitus were the only two primary renal disease categories that seem to predispose patients to myocardial infarction. Shideman[33] found that diabetics who had a high incidence of hypoglycemia and who were undergoing dialysis had a higher incidence of fatal myocardial infarction. All of the patients who died of myocardial infarctions had previous histories of angina and seemed to have more hypotensive than hypertensive episodes during their dialysis procedures. The patients with myocardial infarction averaged 38 years of age while those dialysis patients who survived averaged 32 years of age.

Because of the high incidence of acute myocardial infarction in chronic renal failure, these patients should be informed of cardiovascular symptomatology so they may recognize these symptoms and seek medical attention. Since resuscitation from ventricular fibrillation[34] before arrival at the hospital may decrease morality, personnel concerned with dialysis should have courses in cardiac resuscitation and emergency treatment of cardiac dysrhythmias. The chronic renal patient is already receiving close medical attention and is very familiar with medical terms and medical treatment and does not have the usual apprehension patients have in seeking out physicians for he is routinely contacting physicians with the multiple problems of dialysis. He should have available to him emergency medical phone numbers and facilities where cardiac emergency care is available.

Clinical Presentation

Symptoms of myocardial infarction in the chronic renal patient may be confusing. Early signs of myocardial infarction, such as weakness, easy fatigability, breathlessness, and even hiccups, may be symptoms associated with uremia. Myocardial infarction usually produces retrosternal discomfort lasting more than 15 min, often radiating to the shoulders, arms, neck, or abdomen and not necessarily precipitated by exercise nor relieved by nitroglycerin. The problem is that renal patients may already have had the pain of pericardial disease which may be similar to myocardial ischemic pain and often delays their call for medical attention. Distinguishing between pericardial and myocardial pain is often difficult even for the physician.

Many of the features of myocardial infarction are symptoms which the dialysis patient has frequently. Dizziness or syncope may occur in patients with normal myocardial function who are too rapidly volume depleted; syncope may also occur with dialysis in those patients who already have abnormal myocardial function and who are dependent upon preload and the Starling mechanism to maintain cardiac output. Diaphoresis and palpitations are common during dialysis but also may be an indication of covert myocardial infarction. Dyspnea, paroxysmal nocturnal dyspnea, and orthopnea are routinely present in dialysis patients and might not be taken as symptoms of acute myocardial infarction.

Nausea and vomiting were present in 50 percent of our myocardial infarction patients with chronic renal failure, but may be present without myocardial infarction. Other diseases associated with chronic renal failure, such as esophagitis, cholecystitis, peptic ulcer, pulmonary embolism, dissecting aneurysm, pancreatitis, and arthritis, tend to complicate the historical diagnosis of acute myocardial infarction.

Similarly, physical findings present in chronic renal failure tend to make the diagnosis of acute myocardial infarction difficult. The sallow yellow color of uremia may easily be confused with the ashen pallor of acute myocardial infarction. Likewise, in patients with myocardial infarction, pain often causes increased blood pressure, but the renal failure patient may already be hypertensive and this causes difficulty with therapy. Examination of the retinal fundi will provide clues to the duration of existence of the hypertension. Hypotension, common in myocardial infarction, similarly occurs with dialysis. Tachycardia[35] as well as atrial and ventricular gallops[36] occurring with acute myocardial infarction are almost universal in chronic renal failure. With acute myocardial infarction in chronic renal failure, the significance of gallop rhythm becomes questionable both from a diagnostic and prognostic point of view since their presence usually antecedes the infarct.

Similarly, systolic and diastolic murmurs are more common in chronic renal failure patients.[25,37] The harsh, loud, short duration systolic murmur of chronic uremia could easily be confused with the murmur of acute papillary muscle dysfunction or rupture. Similarly, pericardial friction rubs which are often present in chronic renal failure might be confused with those heard in myocardial infarction. The abnormal cardial apex impulse or ectopic pericardial bulge due to an infarcted area of the myocardium is often already present in chronic renal failure patients. Neck vein distension which may be present in acute myocardial infarction is very often present in the circulatory congestion of chronic renal insufficiency. Most of these patients have long standing hypertension, anemia, acidosis, AV fistulas, and expanded blood volume contributing to the neck vein distension.[38,39] Pleural effusions and rales, signs of pulmonary congestion, are present in a large percentage of patients with chronic renal failure making the diagnosis of pulmonary edema secondary to myocardial infarction difficult. As much as 87 percent of the patients with chest x-rays obtained in chronic renal failure may have signs of congestion.

Laboratory

Electrocardiographic changes of acute myocardial infarction are less specific in the chronic renal failure patient. Del Greco[40] found none of the tracings interpreted before dialysis to be within normal limits. Most common abnormalities were those of T wave and RST segment abnormalities, evidence of left ventricular hypertrophy, and intraventricular conduction defects. After every dialysis, the number of QRS, ST, and T wave changes was diminished by 40 percent, but the number of patterns of left ventricular hypertrophy and strain were doubled. A pattern resembling myocardial infarction was even present in two patients after dialysis, but obscured predialysis. Levine[41] reported four cases with current of injury suggestive of myocardial infarction in predialysis patients not present after dialysis. Arnsdorf[42] reported the electrographic pattern of anteroseptal wall myocardial infarction mimicked by hyperkalemia induced disturbance of impulse conduction and warned of the difficulty in making the diagnosis of acute myocardial infarction in the presence of hyperkalemia.

Enzyme determination of myocardial infarction is also altered in chronic renal failure. Cairns and coworkers[43] report that alterations in plasma volume can change the serial CPK determination. Wesley and others[44] have shown the presence of CPK brain band in the serum of chronic renal disease patients possibly leading to confusion when total CPK is analyzed.

Myocardial scintigraphy with technetium pyrophosphate is used in detecting and sizing acute myocardial infarctions. Janowitz and coworkers[45] showed that there is intense myocardial uptake of Tc-diphosphonate in uremic patients because of secondary hyperparathyroidism and pericarditis. "Super bone scan" occurs because secondary hyperparathyroidism and calcific pericarditis cause increased uptake in the sternal area which is used as the baseline. The readings may be inaccurate and scanning may not be as helpful in the chronic renal patient as in the routine patients with myocardial infarction.

Not all patients with myocardial infarction require hemodynamic measurements. Certain clinical signs may indicate their usefulness. In our own experience, heart failure, ventricular gallop sounds, and rales in the lungs constitute the three most important indications for hemodynamic measurements in myocardial infarction patients. However, in the uremic patient, these signs are almost always present making it mandatory for the uremic patient with suspected myocardial infarction to have hemodynamic measurements.

In the patient with acute myocardial infarction but without renal failure, there is normally a decrease in left ventricular systolic pressure, decrease in maximal rate of rise of pressure, decreased stroke volume, decreased cardiac output, and elevated end-diastolic ventricular pressure. In chronic renal failure, the bedside catheterization varies in that most of the veins in the extremities, and in particular those of the arms, are thrombosed as the result of repeated use for access to the hemodialysis machine. This might even account for the differences in cardiac output since recirculation might occur in peripheral measurements.[46] Kim[47] showed that increased cardiac output was due to an increase in heart rate but normal stroke volume in chronic renal failure (see Chapter 2). Mostert and coworkers[46] found the mean right heart pressures were normal in acute pulmonary edema in chronic renal failure. They pointed out that it was the changing values of continuous cardiac monitoring that are of major importance in following the effects in renal failure rather than the absolute values of the initial measurements itself. Gibson and coworkers[48] postulate that the relative contribution to ultrafiltration in increased capillary permeability to the pathogenesis of pulmonary edema could be assessed by measurement of the pulmonary capillary pressure during an acute attack. They found that the pulmonary vascular pressures were lower than those observed in acute pulmonary edema due to mitral stenosis and left ventricular failure.

Mostert and coworkers[46] also stated that when interstitial pulmonary edema was found at radiographic examination without adventitious sounds in the lungs, and when patients did not have symptomatic signs of failure, expanded blood volume was present. It can be seen, also, that high cardiac output which accompanies chronic renal failure might be confusing in the patient with acute myocardial infarction and low cardiac output. Because of the initial high cardiac output in renal failure, the low cardiac output associated with acute myocardial infarction may be masked and thus the patient may be at greater risk. According to Mostert and coworkers,[46] an expanded volume was the best single sign of circulatory congestion, and they felt that it was the most important single parameter to monitor sequentially in order to determine failure.

Management

Management of the patient with myocardial infarction should be restricted to the coronary care area. The equipment necessary for dialysis should be brought to the unit with the personnel who normally perform the dialysis. Venous and arterial puncture for routine use should be avoided to preserve vessels which are heavily used and especially susceptible to hematoma. After the patient is stable for one week, he may be transferred to the dialysis unit for dialysis. Restriction of sodium to less than 4 gm daily is extremely important to prevent volume expansion and the fluctuations which normally occur between dialysis periods.

Psychological rehabilitation of the chronic renal patient is extremely important, and in our own series 50 percent of our patients with chronic renal failure and acute myocardial infarction has some obvious psychological disturbances as compared to the 10 percent in patients without chronic renal failure. For this reason, the continuity of contact with nephrology team and dialysis technicians is recommended so that depression might be handled by familiar faces.

The monitoring of the patient with myocardial infarction is made more complicated as mentioned above by the fact that the majority of these patients have histories of dysrhythmia, and it is often difficult to determine the acuteness of presenting rhythms. Many of these patients are already on antidysrhythmic medications which makes their use in the treatment of newly developing dysrhythmias even more difficult. When applying hemodynamic measurements to determine therapy for myocardial infarction, it must be remembered that although the patient may have clinical evidence of pulmonary edema, intravascular pressures may be normal and the pulmonary edema would still have to be treated. Although the pulmonary artery end-diastolic pressures may be normal, in such cases pulmonary artery end-diastolic pressures less than 20 may have to be lowered even further in order to reduce the symptoms of pulmonary edema.

Similarly, a single measurement of the cardiac index is not reliable in decisions in which pharmacologic interventions may be made. Clinical findings and symptomatology corresponding to serial changes in hemodynamic measurements must be used more than the absolute measurements. If one finds tachycardia and normal cardiac output in myocardial infarction and chronic renal failure, care should be used with beta blockers since the use of drugs, such as propranolol, might reduce the tachycardia which contributes toward the normal cardiac output. Similarly, if blood pressure is not elevated during acute myocardial infarction with chronic renal failure, hypovolemia and decreased salt intake may be causative. If the blood pressure is elevated, extra care in therapy must be taken for it is usually due to a combination of the intrinsic high blood pressure found in chronic renal failure plus the extra sympathetic discharge associated with myocardial infarction. Separating the contributing causes is almost impossible but necessary since the elevations of blood pressure associated with chronic renal failure usually require larger doses of antihypertensive medications in contrast to the blood pressure rise with myocardial infarction which may need only analgesics. A large number of patients are receiving steroids and their continuation, although possible contributors to increased blood pressure and volume overload, must be maintained.

If pulmonary artery end-diastolic pressure (PAP) is elevated, furosemide may no longer be effective, either by means of decreasing preload or by diuresis. Dialysis is available; however, it must be remembered that peripheral resistance and cardiac work increase during dialysis. If the patient is normovolemic, one must determine if cardiac output would be improved with hemodialysis by determining the volume status of the patient beforehand. If the volume of the patient is increased during the infarction, dialysis would probably improve cardiac output. In a patient with borderline hemodynamic stability, rapid reduction in intravascular volume may have deleterious results, and it is necessary with this patient to make sure priming fluid is used so that volume does not rapidly decrease. Increasing osmolality of the dialyzing fluid can modify the rapidity of the dialysis and avoid embarrassing hemodynamics. The hematocrit should probably be kept above 30 percent as well as it seems better tolerated during this period of cardiovascular instability.

SUMMARY

This chapter has reviewed the process of atherosclerosis and lipid abnormalities which provide the nidus for the development of ischemic heart disease culminating in acute myocardial infarction. The subtleties of diagnosis and treatment of myocardial infarction in patients with ESRD have been discussed. The specific complications of heart failure, arrhythmias, hypertension, and endocarditis are discussed in subsequent chapters.

REFERENCES

1. Lowrie, E.G., Lazarus, J.M., and Mocelin, A.J.: Survival of patients undergoing chronic hemodialysis and renal transplantation. N. Engl. J. Med. 288:863, 1973.
2. Lowrie, E.G., Lazarus, J.M., Hampers, C.L., et al.: Cardiovascular disease in dialysis patients. N. Engl. J. Med. 290:737, 1974.
3. Lindner, A., Charra, B., Sherrard, D.J., et al.: Accelerated atherosclerosis in prolonged maintenance hemodialysis. N. Engl. J. Med. 290:697, 1974.
4. Rostand, S.G., Gretes, J.C., Kirk, K.A., et al.: Ischemic heart disease in patients with uremia undergoing maintenance hemodialysis. Kidney Internat. 16:600, 1979.
5. Nicholls, A.J., Catto, G.R.D., Edward, N., et al.: Accelerated atherosclerosis in long-term dialysis and renal transplant patients: Fact or fiction? Lancet 1:276, 1980.
6. Gordon, T., Castelli, W.P., Hjortland, M., et al.: High density lipoprotein as a protective factor against coronary heart disease. Am. J. Med. 62:707, 1977.
7. Golbourt, U., and Medalie, J.H.: High density lipoprotein cholesterol and incidence of coronary heart disease—the Israeli Ischemic Heart Disease Study. Am. J. Epidemiol. 109(3):296, 1979.
8. Bagdade, J.D., and Albers, J.J.: Plasma high density lipoprotein concentrations in chronic hemodialysis and renal transplantations. N. Engl. J. Med. 296:1436, 1977.

9.   Kaye, J.P., Moorhead, J.F., and Wills, M.R.: Plasma lipids in patients with chronic renal failure. Clin. Chim. Acta 44:301, 1973.

10. Ivels, L.S., Alfred, A.C., and Weil, R.: Hyperlipidemia in adult, pediatric and diabetic renal transplant recipients. Am. J. Med. 64:634, 1978.

11. Bagdade, J.D.: Lipemia, a sequela of chronic renal failure and hemodialysis. Am. J. Clin. Nutrition 21:426, 1968.

12. Bagdade, J.D., Porta, D., Jr., and Bierman, E.L.: Hypertriglyceridemia in metabolic consequence of chronic renal failure. N. Engl. J. Med. 279:191, 1968.

13. Mordasini, R., Frey, F., Floury, W., et al.: Selected deficiency of hepatic triglyceride lipase in uremic patients. N. Engl. J. Med. 297:1362, 1977.

14. Murase, T., Cattran, D.C., Rubinstein, B., et al.: Inhibition of lipoprotein lipase by uremic plasma: A possible cause of hyperglyceridemia. Metabolism 24:1279, 1975.

15. Dombeck, D.H., Lindholm, D.D., and Vieiera, J.A.: Lipid metabolism in uremia and the effects of dialysate glucose and oral androgen therapy. Trans. Am. Soc. Artif. Inter. Organs 19:50, 1973.

16. Yeshurun, D.E., and Gotto, A.M., Jr.: Drug treatment of hyperlipidemia. Am. J. Med. 60:379, 1976.

17. The Coronary Drug Project Research Group: Gall bladder disease as a side-effect of drugs influencing lipid metabolism. N. Engl. J. Med. 296:1187, 1977.

18. Bagdade, J.D.: Atherosclerosis in patients undergoing maintenance hemodialysis. Kidney Internat. 7:370, 1975.

19. Bagdade, J.D., Shantharam, V.V., Sollek, M., et al.: Effects of clofibrate on plasma lipids and high-density lipoprotein levels. Clin. Nephrol. 12:83, 1979.

20. Goldberg, A.B., Applebaum-Bowden, D.M., Bierman, E.L., et al.: Increase in lipoprotein lipase during clofibrate treatment of hypertriglyceridemia in patients on hemodialysis. N. Engl. J. Med. 301:1073, 1979.

21. Gugler, R. Clinical pharmacokinetics of hypolipidaemic drugs. Clin. Pharmacokinet. 3:425, 1978.

22. Bridgmon, J.F., Rosen, S.M., and Thorp, J.M.: Complications during clofibrate treatment of nephrotic syndrome hyperlipoproteinemia. Lancet 2:507, 1972.

23. Langer, T., and Levy, R.I.: Acute muscular syndrome with administration of clofibrate. N. Engl. J. Med. 279:856, 1968.

24. Perez-Garcia, A., Bretro, M., Alvarino, J., et al.: Influence of several factors that intervene in hemodialysis on serum levels of triglycerides and free fatty acids. Clin. Nephrol. 12:14, 1979.

25. Matalon, R., Mousalli, A.R.J., Nidus, B.D., et al.: Functional aortic insufficiency—a feature of renal failure. N. Engl. J. Med. 285:1522, 1971.

26. Schwartz, E.E., and Onesti, G.: The cardiopulmonary manifestations of uremia and renal transplantation. Radiol. Clin. N. Am. 10:569, 1972.

27. Jacobs, C., Aubert, P., and Legrain, M.: Les complications cardio-vasculaires de l'uremic depassee. Ann. Cardiol. Angelol 22:401, 1973.

28. Bauer, G.E.: Modification in the mortality pattern of hypertensive disease: a ten-year prospective. Aust. N.Z. J. Med. 1:4, 1972.

29. Sheil, A.G.R., Stewart, J.H., Johnson, J.R., et al.: Community treatment of end-stages renal failure by dialysis and renal transplantation from cadaver donors. Lancet 2:917, 1969.

30. Report of the National Dialysis Registry (April 1, 1976) Death Analysis: Primary Causes of Death.

31. Mahoney, J.F., Ibels, L., Sheil, R., et al.: Renal transplantation. JAMA 235:2318, 1976.

32. The 12th Report of the Human Renal Transplant Registry. JAMA 233:787, 1975.

33. Shideman, J.R., Buselmeier, T.J., and Kjellstrand, C.M.: Hemodialysis in diabetes. Arch. Intern. Med. 136:1126, 1976.

34. Baum, R., Alverez, H., and Cobb, L.: Survival after resuscitation from out-of-hospital ventricular fibrillation. Circulation 50:1235, 1974.

35. Kim, K.E., Onesti, G., Fernandes, M., et al.: Hemodynamics of hypertension, in Onesti, G., Fernandes, M., and Kim, K.E. (eds.): Regulation of the Blood Pressure by the Central Nervous System. Grune & Stratton, New York, 1976, p. 337.

36. Veda, H., Sakamoto, T., and Sawayama, T.: Clinical phonocardiographic studies of gallop rhythm: report II re-evaluation of kidney gallop. Jap. Heart J. 5(3):201, May 1964.

37. Adam, W.R., Dawborn, J.K., and Rosenbaum, M.: Transient early diastolic murmurs in patients with renal failure. Med. J. Aust. 2:1085, 1970.

38. Kim, K., Onesti, G., and Swartz, C.: Hemodynamics of hypertension in uremia. Kidney Inter. 7(Suppl. 2):155, 1975.

39. Del Greco, F., Simon, N., Roguska, J., et al.: Hemodynamic studies in chronic uremia. Circulation 40:87, 1969.

40. Del Greco, F., and Grumer, H.: Electrolyte and electrocardiographic changes in the course of hemodialysis. Am. J. Cardiol. 9:43, 1962.

41. Levine, H., Wanzer, S., and Merrill, J.P.: Dialyzable currents of injury in potassium intoxication resembling acute myocardial infarction or pericarditis. Circulation 13:29, 1956.

42. Arnsdorf, B.: Electrocardiogram in hyperkalemia. Arch. Intern. Med. 136:1161, 1976.

43. Cairns, J.A., and Klassen, G.A.: The effect of propranolol on canine myocardial CPK distribution space and rate of disappearance. Circulation 56:284, 1977.

44. Wesley, S.A., Byrnes, A., Alter, S., et al.: Presence of creatinine phosphokinase brain bank in the serum of chronic renal disease patients. Clin. Nephrol. 8:345, 1977.

45. Janowitz, W.R., and Serafini, A.N.: Intense myocardial uptake of ^{99m}Tc diphosphonate in a uremic patient with secondary hyperparathyroidism and pericarditis: case report. J. Nuclear Med. 17:896, 1976.

46. Mostert, J.W., Evers, J.L., Hobika, G.H., et al.: The hemodynamic response to chronic renal failure as studied in the azotemic state. Br. J. Anaesth. 42:397, 1970.

47. Kim, K.E., Onesti, G., Neff, M., et al.: Hemodynamic alterations in hypertension of chronic end-stage renal disease, in Onesti, G., Kim, K.E., and Moyer, J.H. (eds.): Hypertension: Mechanisms and Management. Grune & Stratton, New York, 1973, p. 609.

48. Gibson, D.G.: Hemodynamic factors in the development of acute pulmonary edema in renal failure. Lancet 2:1217, 1966.

7

MANAGEMENT OF FLUID RETENTION AND CONGESTIVE HEART FAILURE

LIONEL U. MAILLOUX, M.D.
AND ROBERT T. MOSSEY, M.D.

The addition of the potent diuretics to the medical armamentarium has afforded new approaches for the successful management of significant fluid retention in patients with moderate renal dysfunction (serum creatinine over 3.0 mg/dl). In addition, the renewed interest in peritoneal dialysis and the more recent application of ultrafiltration to these patients have broadened available therapies. Prior to this, these patients presented the clinician with a nearly impossible therapeutic challenge. Often, the pathogenetic mechanism leading to hypervolemia itself stimulates increased tubular reabsorption of sodium, aggravating the underlying disorder. Effectively, utilizing these new modalities requires an understanding of the so-called normal physiology of the abnormal kidney.

PHYSIOLOGIC CONSIDERATIONS

The loss of nephron function that characterizes progressive renal disease produces marked disturbances in both sodium and water metabolism. The maintenance of sodium balance in chronic renal insufficiency requires that the residual nephron populations increase their fractional excretion of sodium. If this were not the case, continual salt and water retention would expand the extracellular fluid space causing hypertension and edema. In addition, since daily sodium intake often varies quite widely, the residual nephrons must somehow still retain the capacity to alter sodium excretion in response to these variations in intake. If this were not the case, the patient with chronic renal disease, in all likelihood, would live his life somewhere between periods of malignant hypertension and shock. Although the factors controlling the increase in fractional sodium excretion are not completely understood, they are in most instances quite effective in maintaining homeostasis.

Through some as yet unknown mechanism, increases in sodium intake are sensed by control centers. Once stimulated, these control centers set into motion a series of events which lead to an increase in total sodium excretion. In the case of the patient with chronic renal insufficiency, this increase in sodium excretion might be mediated by four distinct mechanisms: glomerular filtration rate, peritubular capillary hydrostatic and oncotic pressure, aldosterone, and natriuretic hormone.

First, there could be a substantial increase in single nephron glomerular filtration rate. By increasing the filtered load of sodium while maintaining a fixed tubular reabsorptive capacity, total urinary sodium excretion would rise, a phenomenon which has been documented in experimental animals.[1] This hypothesis, however, has not been documented in man and, even if true, would be unlikely by itself to substantially increase sodium excretion to the degree seen in chronic renal insufficiency. Second, extracellular fluid volume expansion could produce changes in the so-called physical factors surrounding the proximal tubule.[2,3] These changes in the peritubular oncotic and hydrostatic pressures, acting like the Starling forces at the capillary level, could have a marked effect on sodium excretion. For example, by expanding extracellular fluid volume, peritubular hydrostatic pressure is increased and the oncotic pressure decreased. These changes favor back diffusion of sodium into the proximal tubule and increase urinary sodium excretion. Conversely, decreases in the extracellular fluid volume lower hydrostatic pressure and raise oncotic pressure favoring reabsorption of sodium. Third, the increase in fractional sodium excretion could be mediated by changes in aldosterone secretion. Data to support this as a major control factor are lacking. The large increase in fractional sodium excretion seen in chronic renal failure would require almost total suppression of aldosterone production. On the contrary, aldosterone levels in chronic renal failure tend to be elevated.[4] Finally, the increased sodium excretion could be mediated by the production of *natriuretic hormone*. Whether this hormone exists or not has been debated for years. Recent studies, however, tend to confirm the existence of such a substance.[5-7] The magnitude of the natriuresis induced by this substance suggests that it may be the prime factor increasing sodium excretion in chronic renal insufficiency.

Whatever these adaptive mechanisms might be, patients with chronic renal insufficiency demonstrate a well defined maximum excretory rate for sodium.[8] In other words, a patient with stable renal function will demonstrate an upper limit to sodium excretion. If sodium intake exceeds this upper limit, edema and hypertension develop. This limit to sodium excretability varies from individual to individual and is dependent on the nature of the renal disease and the degree of renal impairment. Notably, in any given patient, the upper limit on sodium excretion decreases with progressive nephron loss.

In addition to having an upper limit of sodium excretory capacity, markedly diseased kidneys cannot quickly adapt to abrupt changes in dietary sodium intake.[9] Sodium conservation can be achieved experimentally and in the human only if sodium intake is reduced slowly.[10,11] On the other hand, if sodium intake is abruptly diminished, a negative sodium balance quickly occurs. In other words, a patient with chronic renal failure does not have a true salt losing tendency. Rather, he is unable to rapidly adjust to decreases in sodium intake when compared to the quick sodium retaining response of a person with a normal kidney.

Abnormalities in concentrating and diluting ability are also found in patients with chronic renal insufficiency. They result from the progressive anatomic loss of nephrons, from inhibitors of antidiuretic hormone, and from the constant osmotic diuresis per nephron which occurs in chronic renal insufficiency. As the nephron population diminishes, these factors lead to vasopressin-resistant isosthenuria.[12,13] The result is that the daily urinary volume is relatively fixed and determined by the relationship of the approximately 600 mOsm of solute to be excreted and the maximum urine osmolality. To illustrate, if maximum urinary osmolality is 300 mOsm/L, 2L/day will be necessary to maintain solute balance. In the otherwise normal, alert, and unrestricted patient with chronic renal failure, normal thirst mechanisms will assure an adequate fluid intake to prevent dehydration. However, when consciousness is impaired or fluid restricted, the patient is unable to further concentrate his urine and a negative water balance quickly develops.

Although diluting ability is better preserved than concentrating ability, an upper limit on free water excretion can be demonstrated in most patients with chronic renal insufficiency.[14] Clinically, this observation rarely poses a problem except when there is an acute deterioration of renal function and oral intake is not decreased or if the old adage of "forcing fluids to flush the kidney" is employed. Under these circumstances, water retention and a progressive dilutional state of life threatening proportions can develop.

Loss of concentrating ability to a major extent and diluting ability to a lesser extent lead to a relatively fixed minimal urinary output necessary to maintain osmotic balance and place an upper limit on water excretion. Thus, if fluid intake falls below the minimal urinary output dictated by the patient's osmotic needs, progressive hemoconcentration will occur;

whereas if the upper limit on free water excretion is exceeded, hemodilution will occur.

CLINICAL IMPLICATIONS

Four questions, therefore, are suggested by the physiologic factors discussed above. First, has the patient's salt intake exceeded his maximum excretory ability? Second, has there been a significant change in renal function to account for excessive sodium and water retention? Third, has there been a change in the patient's fluid intake or urinary output to explain problems of hemodilution or hemoconcentration? Fourth, are there any superimposed factors interfering with the diseased kidney's normal sodium control mechanisms? Superimposed illnesses such as the nephrotic syndrome, congestive heart failure, and cirrhosis of the liver can affect the physical factors surrounding the proximal tubule and markedly decrease maximum urinary sodium excretion. Similarly, a marked decrease in sodium intake will reduce urinary sodium excretion by decreasing the single nephron glomerular filtration rate. Commonly used drugs, such as antihypertensives and anti-inflammatory agents, can adversely affect the glomerular filtration rate or the physical factors surrounding the proximal tubule and increase sodium reabsorption (Table 1). The proper assessment of the renal failure patient, then, depends on an understanding of the physiologic mechanisms by which the diseased kidneys still endeavor to maintain the body integrity. These adaptations are remarkably successful through a wide range of renal dysfunction; but eventually they fail, leading to fluid retention. At this point, careful therapeutic intervention becomes necessary to assist the kidney to maintain homeostasis.

THERAPY

General Measures

The same therapeutic guidelines that are used in other patients with hypervolemia are applied to patients with moderate renal insufficiency (Table 2).

The initial aim should be to establish the cause and severity of hypervolemia before embarking on a potentially dangerous treatment plan. This will enable the treating physician to initiate appropriate therpy. The therapeutic plan will differ considerably whether the patient has underlying heart disease and congestive heart failure or fluid overload superimposed on chronic renal disease.

The early morning daily weight after the patient has urinated will give

TABLE 1. Commonly used antidiuretic drugs

Salicylates	Vincristine
Indomethacin	Cyclophosphamide
Phenylbutazone	Carbamazapine
Chlorpropamide	Minoxidil
Clofibrate	

more meaningful information about salt and water balance than any other single test. Fluctuations in daily weight are important guidelines for the physician to follow.

Quantitation of the patient's daily sodium intake plays a vital role in the management plan. This frequently requires a coordinated effort between the physician, nurse, and dietitian. If the patient is ambulatory, requesting three consecutive days' dietary record (including at least one weekend day) will accomplish the same objective. During this period, the daily urinary volume and sodium excretion should be determined. If weight increases are noted, the sodium intake can then be gradually decreased below the daily output. If weight loss is noted, the sodium intake may be slowly increased. This is especially important in patients who may have relative sodium losing diseases, for example, interstitial nephritis, polycystic kidney disease, or medullary cystic kidney disease. Acute and strict sodium restriction is contraindicated in these disorders. Medications which can have a profound effect on renal sodium excretion (Table 1) should be avoided unless they are considered absolutely necessary.

TABLE 2. Therapy of hypervolemia in patients with moderate to severe renal insufficiency

A. General Measures
   Daily weight
   Dietary history
   Sodium restriction
   Assessment of urgency of therapy
   Bed rest
   Frequent renal function tests
B. Digitalis, if indicated
C. Diuretics
D. Peritoneal dialysis*
E. Ultrafiltration*

*These measures are reserved for refractory fluid overload.

Maintenance of renal blood flow and glomerular filtration rate while reducing hypervolemia is the primary goal of therapy. This is sometimes difficult to achieve. During therapy, frequent determinations of the serum creatinine and serum urea nitrogen are necessary to gauge the effects of therapy on renal function. Indeed, changes in these parameters during treatment may require cessation of therapy or the addition of other therapeutic modalities. For example, in the treatment of severe nephrotic syndrome, the difference between adequate and inadequate renal perfusion is small. A minimal diuresis may precipitate profound decrease in the effective circulating blood volume and shock can ensue dramatically. Supporting the blood volume with salt-poor albumin may be necessary while diuresing some nephrotic patients, despite the apparent contradiction that this presents. Controlling nephrotic edema is not an emergent medical problem and should be treated gently.

On the other hand, the patient with congestive heart failure may require the addition of other therapeutic modalities. In these patients, digitalization and preload and afterload reduction may stabilize and/or improve deteriorating renal function. The pharmacokinetics and proper use of digitalis preparations are presented in Chapter 3.

Diuretics

Diuretics are reserved for those clinical situations that have not responded to the simpler therapeutic modalities. Even a minimal decrease in circulating blood volume may cause a stable patient with chronic renal insufficiency to develop progressive renal failure. When this is noted, the offending agents must be discontinued and the patient slowly rehydrated in an attempt to stabilize renal function. These drugs should not be prescribed unless renal function can be followed closely.

Organomercurials should be noted because of their historical status and viewed with respect. They are effective in patients with midly decreased glomerular filtration rates and in the face of metabolic acidosis.[15,16] Their use is limited by their nephrotoxicity.[17,18] These drugs have been completely replaced by newer, more potent, and more versatile diuretics.

Since their introduction in the 1950's, the thiazides have become the most widely used diuretics. The thiazides are effective in controlling hypertension and causing a diuresis in patients with mildly impaired renal function. As the glomerular filtration rate decreases further, thiazide action is less predictable. When the serum creatinine reaches a level of 3.0 to 3.5 mg/dl thiazides are rarely of therapeutic value. In addition, they may be ineffective in the presence of hypoalbuminemia of the nephrotic syndrome even with a glomerular filtration rate only reduced to 50 or 60 ml/min.

Ethacrynic acid and furosemide were the first diuretics that proved to be effective in the treatment of overhydration in renal impairment.[19-23] They are totally different compounds structurally, yet their site and mode of action are similar affecting active chloride transport in the ascending limb of the loop of Henle.[25, 26] Furosemide and ethacrynic acid are actively secreted through the tubular cell by the aryl acid pumps into the urine of the proximal tubule.[27] These drugs are more active from the urinary side of the tubule than the peritubular surface. Hook and Williamson have shown that probenecid, an aryl acid transport inhibitor, can block the diuresis caused by furosemide in the dog.[28] Unlike the thiazides, their effectiveness extends to patients with markedly impaired renal function, and they are often effective in the presence of the hypoalbuminemia of severe nephrotic syndrome.[19]

Proper dosage is important in achieving an effective diuresis with the loop diuretics (Table 3). The amount of drug to achieve diuresis must exceed a threshold dose that increases as renal function declines. This dose may be given as a single daily dose or may be repeated several times daily. This threshold dose may depend upon proximal tubular secretion which might be depressed by the increased levels of organic acids in the blood. Once the threshold dose has been determined, a significant increase in diuresis will occur with relatively small increments in dosage. The total daily dose of furosemide may range from 80 to 1000 mg, while ethacrynic acid has a narrower dose range of 50 to 300 mg. If diuretic induced hypokalemia becomes a problem, potassium chloride supplementation should be given carefully with frequent monitoring of the serum potassium level. Spironolactone, triamterene, and amiloride are contraindicated in patients with serum creatinine levels above 3 mg/dl. The combination of renal insufficiency, potassium chloride supplementation, and potassium retaining diuretics should be avoided because it may result in lethal hyperkalemia.

Intravenous adminstration of furosemide and ethacrynic acid may be used in place of oral medications. The initial intravenous doses of

TABLE 3. Useful diuretics in renal insufficiency

Drug	Daily Dose Range	Site of Action
Furosemide	80 mg to 1000 mg	Loop of Henle ? proximal tubule at high dose
Ethacrynic acid	50 mg to 300 mg	Loop of Henle
Metolazone	5 mg to 50 mg	Cortical diluting site ? proximal tubule at high dose

furosemide and ethacrynic acid need not be as large as the oral dose. One should expect a longer lasting diuresis in patients with renal insufficiency rather than the three to four hour duration seen in patients with relatively normal renal function. The parenteral use of the potent diuretics should be reserved for medical emergencies and patients who cannot take oral medications. The major hazard in the use of both these drugs is ototoxicity. Furosemide may cause transient tinnitus and deafness; the latter may be longer lasting after exceedingly large intravenous doses. In addition, there has been a suggestion that furosemide may rarely cause interstitial nephritis that may further complicate the underlying renal disorder. Permanent deafness has been described with both oral and intravenous ethacrynic acid in patients with renal failure.

Metolazone, which was introduced in this country in the mid-1970s, is a useful diuretic in these patients.[29] Although not as potent as the loop diuretics, it is more useful than the thiazides. It may be given in daily doses up to 50 mg and is relatively long acting. It is especially useful in patients with edema that is seemingly refractory to furosemide.[30] The addition of metolazone to furosemide in even modest doses results in a greater diuresis than one would expect from either drug alone. This synergy with furosemide, which has been described in uncontrolled studies, may be of tremendous clinical benefit.[31] This combination has been effective in several patients with anasarca, nephrotic syndrome, serum albumins as low as 0.9 gm/100 ml, and diminished creatinine clearances and whose edema had been refractory to large doses of furosemide averaging 480 mg per day.[32] Striking diureses and weight losses have been seen in 5 patients with so-called refractory edema, renal insufficiency, and high doses of furosemide up to 720 mg (Fig. 1). After 15 mg of metolazone, there was such a prompt diuresis that hospitalization was required in 3 of these patients for hypovolemic shock and severe electrolyte abnormalities. If metolazone is added to furosemide, the dose of furosemide should be halved and no more than 10 mg of metolazone prescribed initially. Frequent weights and electrolyte determinations should be obtained and monitored during the first 72 hours. The loop diuretics and metolazone allow the physician to treat many patients who previously would have been unmanageable. These potent diuretics are not without hazard, but if the patient is followed closely, they may be used safely even at high doses.

Peritoneal Dialysis and Ultrafiltration

Recently, the therapy of severe congestive heart failure has markedly improved prolonging the life of nearly terminal patients. These patients frequently have a degree of intrinsic renal disease and associated

ENHANCED WEIGHT LOSS AFTER THE ADDITION OF METOLAZONE

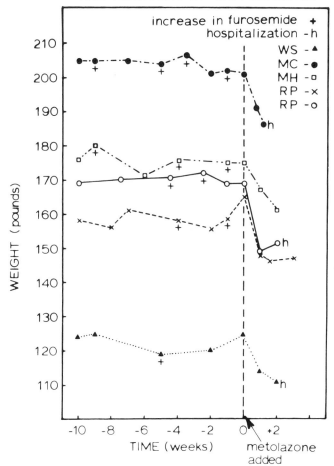

FIGURE 1. A prompt weight loss in noted in 5 patients after the addition of metolazone to furosemide.

nephrosclerosis. This renal disease in itself may not result in massive fluid retention; but because the kidneys are poorly perfused from a diminished cardiac output, their ability to function is markedly impaired. The diminished renal perfusion decreases effective renal blood flow altering the physical factors surrounding the proximal tubule. Ultimately, as the patient's status continues to deteriorate, these factors promote further proximal salt and water retention, reducing distal sodium delivery so that no diuretic response can be achieved. Clinically, this is manifested by an isosthenuric urine with little or no sodium. These patients now require alternate modes of therapy to relieve them of their fluid burden.

The previous use of chronic high dose diuretics has often resulted in severe prerenal azotemia, electrolyte abnormalities, and digitoxic arrhythmias further complicating their medical management. In addition, the kidneys no longer respond to medical therapy. There are two effective mechanical procedures available for removing excess fluid—peritoneal dialysis and ultrafiltration. Peritoneal dialysis has been applied widely for the treatment of acute and chronic renal failure utilizing the peritoneal membrane to remove waste products[33,35] and excess fluids.[36-39] The ability to remove large volumes of fluid has been repeatedly demonstrated in patients undergoing dialysis for uremia. Surprisingly, although hypertonic peritoneal dialysis has a capacity to induce rapid and marked negative fluid balances, this modality has been infrequently utilized to treat severe hypervolemia. Fluid can be readily removed by dialyzing the patient with hypertonic (4.25 percent dextrose) solutions.

Using peritoneal dialysis, negative fluid balances of 12 to 14 L may be achieved within 16 hr.[38] The dialysate that is removed contains mainly water, but there is enough solute so that significant decreases in plasma urea and creatinine levels may be achieved. In addition, metabolic and electrolyte abnormalities, if present, will be corrected rapidly by peritoneal dialysis. Hypotension and shock may ensue if fluid removal is too rapid from patients with such severe congestive heat failure. Paradoxically, the slow removal of fluid may increase the blood pressure and other hemodynamic parameters. Response to diuretics may even be restored after peritoneal dialysis.[39] The reason for this phenomenon is unclear, but may be related to the improved cardiac hemodynamics seen after relief of severe fluid overload.[38] Because peritoneal dialysis may be used in unstable patients, this procedure requires great expertise, constant supervision, and should not be undertaken lightly.

Recently, another technique for fluid removal arising from observations made in chronic hemodialysis may prove to be effective and is being studied extensively. In addition to dialysis, the currently used hemodialyzers cause fluid removal. By optimizing the technical conditions, one may maximize such fluid removal or ultrafiltration with minimal dialysis (Fig. 2).[40]

When a patient's blood is pumped past one side of a dialysis membrane of the same type used for hemodialysis and vacuum pressure is applied to the other side of the dialysis membrane, a plasma ultrafiltrate can be produced.[41-44] This simple procedure permits the direct removal of fluid from the circulation. The amount and rate of fluid

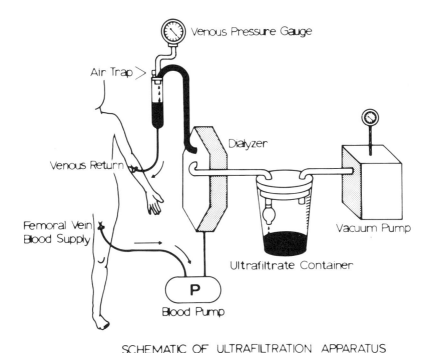

SCHEMATIC OF ULTRAFILTRATION APPARATUS

FIGURE 2. A diagram of the equipment required for ultrafiltration. Note that a vacuum pump is connected to a dialysate port on the dialyzer. No dialysate bathes the dialyzer membrane.

removal is predictable and proportional to the vacuum pressure applied to the membrane and the fluid pressure across the membrane (transmembrane pressure). For each dialyzer, there is an ultrafiltration coefficient that allows the clinician to calculate expected fluid removal rates (Table 4). The ultrafiltrate contains mainly water and solute in the same concentration as in plasma. Serum electrolytes do not change. Up to 4000 ml can be removed by ultrafiltration within 90 to 120 min. without producing untoward symptoms. An example of ultrafiltration is presented in Table 5. This lack of untoward symptoms has been attributed to the fact that ultrafiltration does not alter serum osmolality.[40,45] As plasma volume falls, extracellular fluid shifts into the intravascular compartments and intracellular fluid then moves into the extracellular fluid space to maintain the circulating plasma volume.[41]

The maintenance of plasma volume without alteration of osmolality makes ultrafiltration an ideal adjunct therapy for refractory edema and severe congestive heart failure in patients with renal insufficiency. The time required for several therapies is minimal. Patients tolerate the pro-

TABLE 4. Ultrafiltration coefficients of common dialyzers

Dialyzer	Coefficient ml fluid ultrafiltered/ mm* Hg transmembrane pressure/hour
C-Dak 1.3 m²†	1.5
C-Dak 1.8 m²	2.0
C-Dak 2.5 m²	3.0
Gambro-Lundia Major 11.5 u‡ 1.36 m²	7.0
Gambro-Lundia Plate 11.5 u 1.0 m²	4.0
Gambro-Lundia Plate 17 u 1.0 m²	2.5
Tri-Ex I	4.0
Travenol CF 1200	2.5
Travenol CF 1500	4.0

*For example: using a Gambro-Lundia plate, 11.5 u 1.0 m² and a total transmembrane pressure of 200 mm Hg, optimally one could expect to remove 800 ml of fluid in 1 hr (4 × 200 × 1).
† m² = square meters of surface area.
‡ u = micron thickness of membrane.

cedure quite well despite their severe heart disease. Because an adequate blood flow is required, cannulation of large blood vessels (femoral veins) or the use of an already present arteriovenous fistula is necessary for ultrafiltration. This mode of therapy should be done only by a trained dialysis staff. As in peritoneal dialysis, if fluid removal is achieved slowly, the blood pressure may increase as cardiac output increases. Hypotension may be encountered on occasion. If there are severe electrolyte abnormalities, hemodialysis can be performed after ultrafiltration.

SUMMARY

Increased understanding of the physiologic adaptations ocurring in the diseased kidney has resulted in marked improvement in the care of previously unmanageable patients with severe congestive heart failure and renal insufficiency. Rational therapeutic decisions and proper use of such drugs as furosemide, ethacrynic acid, and metolazone can now be based on sound physiologic principles. Peritoneal dialysis and ultrafiltration have recently been used for the mechanical relief of hypervolemia and electrolyte imbalances. These therapies have also resulted from greater understanding about the renal mechanisms involved.

TABLE 5. Example of ultrafiltration

Pt. J.V.: Severe congestive heart failure, anasarca, aortic and mitral valve disease, coronary artery disease, moderate renal insufficiency (serum creatinine 3.8 mg/100 ml), and unresponsive to furosemide.

Dialyzer: Gambro 11.5 u 1.0 m² (ultrafiltration coefficient 4.0)

Procedure: Femoral venipuncture for blood supply; cephalic venous return.

Time	BP (mm/Hg)	P	Dialyzer blood flow (ml/min)	Transmembrane pressure (mm/Hg)	Pulmonary diastolic pressure (mm/Hg)	Fluid removed (ml)
0	120/90	92	-	-	21	0
15	112/98	98	110	300	21	
30	104/88	94	110	525	19	700
45	100/90		102	575	18	
60	130/78	100	110	550	17	1550
90	150/90	86	160	400	16	
120	170/	80	160	400	16	3000

REFERENCES

1. Liebowitz, H., Purkerson, M.L., Sugita, M., et al.: GFR per nephron and per kidney in the chronically diseased (pyelonephritic) kidney of the rat. Am. J. Physiol. 217:853, 1969.
2. Martino, J.A., and Earley, L.E.: Demonstration of a role of physical factors as determinants of the natriuretic response to volume expansion. J. Clin. Invest. 46:1963, 1967.
3. Brenner, B.M., Falchuk, N.H., Heimowitz, R.I., et al.: The relationship between peritubular capillary protein concentration and fluid reabsorption by the renal proximal tubule. J. Clin. Invest. 48:1519, 1969.
4. Cope, C.L., and Pearson, J.: Aldosterone secretion in severe renal failure. Clin. Sci. 25:331, 1963.
5. Gonick, H.C., and Saldanka, L.E.: A natriuretic principle derived from kidney tissue of volume expanded rats. J. Clin. Invest. 56:247,1975.
6. Kaplan, M.A., Bourgoignie, T.J., Rosecan, J., et al.: The effects of the natriuretic factor from uremic urine on sodium transport, water and electrolyte content, and pyruvate oxidation by the isolated toad bladder. J. Clin. Invest. 53:1568, 1974.
7. Weber, H., Bourgoignie, J., and Bricker, N.S.: Effects of the natriuretic serum fraction on proximal tubular sodium reabsorption. Am. J. Physiol. 226:419, 1974.
8. Bricker, N.S., Klahr, S., Liebowitz, H., et al.: Renal function in chronic renal disease. Medicine (Baltimore) 44:263, 1965.
9. Coleman, H.J., Arias, M., Carter, N.W., et al.: The mechanism of salt wastage in chronic renal disease. J. Clin. Invest. 45:1116, 1966.
10. Schmidt, R.W., Bourgoignie, T.J., and Bricker, N.S.: On the adaptation in sodium excretion in chronic uremia. The effects of 'proportional reduction' of sodium intake. J. Clin. Invest. 53:1736, 1974.
11. Danovitch, G.M., Bourgoignie, J., and Bricker, N.S.: Reversibility of the "salt losing" tendency of chronic renal failure. N. Engl. J. Med. 296:14, 1977.
12. Tannen, R.L., Regal, E.M., Dunn, M.J., et al.: Vasopressin-resistant hyposthenuria in advanced chronic renal disease. N. Engl. J. Med. 280:1135, 1965.
13. Holliday, M.A., Egan, T.J., Morris, C.R., et al.: Pitressin-resistant hyposthnuria in chronic renal disease. Am. J. Med. 42:378, 1967.
14. Kleeman, C.R., Adams, D.A., and Maxwell, M.H.: An evaluation of maximal water diuresis in chronic renal disease: I. normal solute intake. J. Lab. Clin. Med. 58:169, 1961.
15. Cafruny, E.J.: The site and mechanism of action of mercurial diuretics. Pharmacol. Rev. 20:89, 1968.
16. Burg, M., Green, N.: Effect of mersalyl on the thick ascending limb of Henle's loop. Kidney Inter. 4:245, 1973.
17. Freeman, R.B., Maher, J.F., Schreiner, G.E., et al.: Renal tubular necrosis due to nephrotoxicity of organic mercurial diuretics. Ann. Intern. Med. 60:242, 1962.
18. Avram, M.M., Lipner, H.I., and Gan, A.C.: Medical nephrectomy. The use of metallic salts for the control of massive proteinuria in the nephrotic syndrome. Trans. Amer. Soc. Artif. Intern. Organs 22:431, 1976.
19. Muth, R.: Diuretic properties of furosemide in renal disease. Ann. Intern. Med. 69:249, 1968.
20. Gregory, L.F., Durrett, R.R., Robinson, R.R., et al.: The short term effect of furosemide on electrolyte and water excretion in patients with severe renal disease. Arch. Intern. Med. 125:69, 1970.

21. Fairley, K.F., and Laver M.: High dose furosemide in chronic renal failure. Postgrad. Med. J. 47:40, 1971 (Suppl.).

22. Brennan, L.B., and Ebrahami, A.: Experience with furosemide in renal disease. Proc. Soc. Exp. Biol. Med. 118:333, 1965.

23. Maher, J.F., and Schreiner, G.E.: Studies on ethacrynic acid in patients with refractory edema. Ann. Intern. Med. 62:15, 1965.

24. Laragh, J.H., Cannon, P.J., Stason, W.B., et al.: Physiologic and clinical observations on furosemide and ethacrynic acid. Ann. NY Acad. Sci. 139:453,1966.

25. Goldberg, M.: Ethacrynic acid: site and mode of action. Ann. NY Acad. Sci. 139:443, 1966.

26. Bowman, R.H.: Renal secretion of S^{35}-furosemide and its depression by albumin binding. Am. J. Physiol. 229:93, 1975.

27. Burg, M., and Stoner, L.: Renal tubular chloride transport and the mode of action of some diuretics. Ann. Rev. Physiol. 38:37, 1976.

28. Hook, J.B., and Williamson, H.E.: Influence of probenecid and alterations in acid–base balance of the saluretic activity of furosemide. J. Pharmacol. Exper. Ther. 149:404, 1965.

29. Paton, R.R., and Kane, R.E.: Long-term diuretic therapy with metolazone in renal failure and the nephrotic syndrome. J. Clin. Pharmacol. 17:243, 1977.

30. Epstein, M., Lipp, B.A., Hoffman, D.S., et al.: Potentiation of furosemide by metolazone in refractory edema. Curr. Therap. Res. 21:656, 1977.

31. Gunstone, R.F., Wing, A.J., Shane, H.G.P., et al.: Clinical experience with metolazone in fifty–two african patients: synergy with furosemide. Postgrad. Med. J. 47:789, 1971.

32. Friedman, E.A.: Personal communication.

33. Grollman, A., Turner, L.B., and McLean, J.A.: Intermittent peritoneal lavage in nephrectomized dogs and its application to the human being. Arch. Intern. Med. 87:379. 1951.

34. Maxwell, M.H., Rockney, R.E., and Kleeman, C.R.: Peritoneal dialysis — technique and application. JAMA 176:917, 1959.

35. Shear, L., Swartz, C., Shinaberger, J.A., et al.: Kinetics of peritoneal fluid absorption in adult man. N. Engl. J. Med. 272:123, 1965.

36. Schmierson, S.J.: Continuous peritoneal irrigation in the treatment of intractable edema of cardiac origin. Am. J. Med. Sci. 218:76, 1949.

37. Bertrand, E., and Guerin, J.: Peritoneal dialysis with glucose in the irreducible edemas of cardiac patients. Med. Trop. 21:603, 1961.

38. Mailloux, L.U., Swartz, C.D., Onesti, G., et al.: Peritoneal dialysis for refractory congestive heart failure. JAMA 199:873, 1967.

39. Rae, A.I., and Hopper, J.: Removal of refractory edema fluid by peritoneal dialysis. Br. J. Urol. 40:336, 1968.

40. Ing., J.S., Ashbach, D.L., and Kanter, A.: Fluid removal with negative pressure hydrostatic ultrafiltration using a partial vacuum. Nephron 14:451, 1975.

41. Bergstrom, J., Asaba, H., Furest, P., et al.: Dialysis, ultrafiltration, and blood pressure. Proc. Eur. Dial. Transplant Assoc. 13:293, 1976.

42. Bergstrom, J.: Ultrafiltration without dialysis for removal of fluid and solutes in uremia. Clin. Nephrol. 9:156, 1978.

43. Henderson, L.W., Livoti, L., Ford, C., et al.: Clinical experience with intermittent hemodiafiltration. Trans. Am. Soc. Artif. Intern. Organs. 19:119, 1973.

44. Silverstein, M.D., Ford, C.A., Lysaght, M., et al.: Response to rapid removal of intermediate molecular weight solutes in uremic man. Trans. Am. Soc. Artif. Intern. Organs 20:64, 1974.

45. Shinaberger, J.A.: Dialysis. Cur. Nephrol. 1:314, 1977.

8

CARDIAC ARRHYTHMIAS IN CHRONIC RENAL FAILURE

GARY J. ANDERSON, M.D.

DISTURBANCES OF CARDIAC RHYTHM AND CONDUCTION IN RENAL FAILURE

Disturbances of cardiac rhythm and conduction are frequently encountered in patients with renal disease (see Chapters 1 and 6). However, arrhythmias and abnormal conduction may reflect an underlying pathologic process but are not to be considered specific or diagnostic. Moreover, cardiac rhythm and conduction are affected by noncardiac and humoral factors such as serum electrolytes, drugs, and metabolites. It follows, then, that the pathophysiologic processes that are operative to induce an arrhythmia may represent the expression of one or all of these factors acting in concert. This emphasizes the concept that there exists no pathognomonic arrhythmia or conduction disturbance. The clinician confronted by an arrhythmia must consider the pathologic processes involving the heart, either primary or secondary, the electrolyte and metabolic status, and the drug programs of each patient.

Because of this complex interaction of primary or secondary myocardial involvement by a pathologic process and the extrinsic arrhythmogenic stimuli, it is difficult to categorize arrhythmias as to their specific etiology. Similarly it is impossible to "weigh" each contributing factor and analyze the arrhythmia according to its *most important* precipitating factor as this is often obscure. Needless to say, the clinician will not be able to sort out the many factors with precision, but will be armed with the knowledge of the potential synergism of several factors. For instance, chronic renal failure is associated with an increased extracellular volume and hypertension both of which lead to disturbed myocardial function and may be arrhythmogenic. The concomitant acidosis and hyperkalemia are also arrhythmogenic and may act synergistically with the aforementioned factors. When confronted by altered conduction or an arrhythmia, the clinician will not be able to deduce the arrhythmogenic stimulus since it is most likely multifactorial. On the other hand, it is still plausible to invoke more specific precipitating factors eliciting arrhythmias when they occur acutely and subside with correction of the specific abnormality.

ABNORMALITIES OF CONDUCTION AND RHYTHM DUE TO PRIMARY MYOCARDIAL INVOLVEMENT

For the sake of purity of definition, the term "primary" is misleading and is used in the context of abnormalities of conduction and rhythm due to pathophysiologic alteration of the myocardium, although they are obviously "secondary" to the chronic renal disease.

Metastatic calcification has been observed in chronic renal failure[1,2] and may involve the working myocardium, the coronary arteries, or the specialized conduction system of the heart. When the specialized conducting system is involved, there is often concomitant calcification of the interventricular septum. Metastatic calcification of the specialized conducting system is electrocardiographically evident by altered conduction showing first degree AV block or bundle branch block. Terman[2] observed that 2 of 6 patients with metastatic calcification of the specialized conduction system developed complete heart block. Of interest, 2 of these patients died suddenly at home, presumably of cardiac arrhythmias.

The consideration of primary cardiovascular disease in renal failure must include those diseases which produce primary renal and myocardial disease such as scleroderma and polyarteritis nodosa. Table 1 lists these diseases and their pathologic and clinical counterparts are considered elsewhere in this text (Chapter 1). Myocardial involvement in these diseases varies and both arrhythmias and conduction defects are not uncommon. Unfortunately, the observed arrhythmias and patterns are not specific and should not be considered diagnostic although bundle branch block is more common in myopathies producing sclerosis of the myocardium. Table 2 reviews some of the disturbances of rhythm and conduction observed in several of the cardiomyopathies associated with renal involvement. Since primary myocardial disease is often slow in onset, progressive abnormalities of conduction may appear. First degree heart block, bundle branch block, and intraventricular conduction defects may develop early, and progression of the myocardial disease is

TABLE 1. The primary cardiovascular diseases in renal failure

1. Scleroderma	8. Rheumatoid arthritis
2. Polyarteritis nodosa	9. Generalized Schwartzman reaction
3. Systemic lupus erythmatosus	10. Thrombotic thrombocytopenic
4. Amyloidosis	purpura
5. Wegener's granulomatosis	11. Endotoxinemia
6. Fabry's disease	12. Actue glomerulonephritis
7. Primary oxalosis	12. "Myopathy" of chronic renal
	failure

associated with progression of the conduction abnormalities. Deterioration of the cardiac function in any of these diseases precipitates ventricular arrhythmias which often are refractory to conventional therapeutic agents, especially in the presence of end-stage disease. These arrhythmias may respond to the judicious administration of digitalis. It has also been shown that chronic renal failure may be associated with accelerated atherogenesis and coronary artery disease.[3] It is therefore not surprising to find the conduction abnormalities and ventricular tachyarrhythmias commonly encountered in coronary artery disease in chronic renal failure also, even when clinical manifestations of coronary disease are few.

SECONDARY CAUSES OF ARRHYTHMIAS AND CONDUCTION DEFECTS

Digitalis administration in patients with chronic renal disease is often avoided, if possible, because of the high incidence of digitalis intoxication and because most instances of heart failure are related to volume overload (Chapter 7). Moreover, in patients on dialysis, digitalis is found in only trace amounts in the dialysate.[20] The electrocardiographic manifestations of digitalis intoxication are many and are summarized in Table 3.

Sinus bradycardia and sinus tachycardia are both common. Sinus arrest and sinoatrial (SA) block are considered uncommon. However, SA block is probably common but only infrequently recognized. Cases of sinus bradycardia exist which are due to 2:1 SA block but are unrecognized. The diagnosis of these SA arrhythmias is difficult and long rhythm strips are required to demonstrate the transition of 2:1 block to some other conduction pattern such as 3:2 or 4:3 thereby permitting analysis of the arrhythmias. Of the atrial arrhythmias in digitalis toxicity, paroxysmal atrial tachycardia (PAT) is common, more often in association with AV block showing a fixed multiple such as 2:1 or 4:1 or as Wenckebach AV

TABLE 2. Rhythm and conduction disturbances in cardiomyopathy with renal involvement

Disease entity	References	Arrhythmias				Conduction Disturbances			
		SA	Atrial	AV	Vent	SA	AV	BBB	Vent
Scleroderma	4-6	+	+++	+++	+++	0	++	+++	0
Polyarteritis nodosa	7-8	0	+	+	++	0	+	++	+
Systemic lupus erythematosus	9-11	0	+	+	+	0	+	+	0
Amyloidosis	12-14	++	+	+	+	+	+++	++++	+++
Fabry's disease	15-16	+	+	0	0	+	+	+++	+++
Rheumatoid arthritis	17-19	0	++	+	+	0	+++	++++	0

0 = No reports or incidence unknown
+ = Rare
++ = Occasional
+++ = Common

SA = Sinoatrial
AV = Atrioventricular
Vent = Ventricular
BBB = Bundle branch block

TABLE 3. ECG manifestations
of digitalis intoxication

Sinus arrhythmias	5–12%
Atrial arrhythmias	20–30%
AV block	30–40%
Junctional arrhythmias	5–10%
Ventricular arrhythmias	60–85%

block and this does not permit the clinician to exclude digitalis as the etiology. Atrial fibrillation is probably one of the more common arrhythmias seen in digitalis intoxication. This arrhythmia arises subsequent to atrial premature beats falling on the vulnerable phase of atria leading to atrial fibrillation. Most often the ventricular response is slow and this arrhythmia will convert to sinus rhythm after digitalis is discontinued.

Ventricular arrhythmias are predominantly coupled premature systoles, often in a bigeminal fashion, or they may be multiform. While the incidence of this arrhythmia is high and not infrequently produces ventricular tachycardia, the progression to ventricular fibrillation is uncommon.

A practical consideration is why should dialysis precipitate digitalis induced arrhythmias? The two primary mechanisms deal with dialysis induced changes in K^+ and Ca^{++}. Potassium is a competitive inhibitor of digitalis binding to cardiac (and noncardiac) sodium-potassium ATPase. When K^+ is elevated it significantly reduces the binding rate of digitalis to Na^+-K^+ ATPase.[21,22] Similarly, when K^+ is reduced, digitalis binding rates are accelerated. Although beyond the scope of this chapter, digitalis induces abnormal cardiac rhythms by altering the conducting properties of the heart as well as by accelerating or inducing abnormal automaticity.[23,24] A reduction in serum K^+, therefore, would initiate or aggravate an arrhythmia by 1) enhancing digitalis binding to membrane sites and 2) a direct membrane effect of reduced extracellular K^+. Reduced K^+_o also increases automaticity or unmasks it, thereby, potentiating the arrhythmogenic stimulus of cardiac glycosides. Calcium is also known to mediate arrhythmias in digitalis toxicity.[25] It has been long known that digitalis and hypercalcemia are synergistic and that low Ca^{++} is associated with digitalis tolerance and high Ca^{++} with digitalis sensitivity. This is consistent with recent observations showing that digitalis exposure to Purkinje fibers induces "delayed after-depolarizations" or low amplitude potentials after phase 3 of the action potential.[26] These transient "bumps" in membrane potential are directly related to Ca^{++} and are considered to represent a mechanism for ventricular arrhythmias.

Thus, the combined sensitivity of the heart to acidosis, digitalis, and increasing Ca^{++} during dialysis sets an ideal milieu for the development of cardiac arrhythmias. Although the shift in Ca^{++} in dialyzed patients is not great (0.5 mg%),[27] it may often be sufficient to induce digitalis toxic arrhythmias.

The appearance of digitalis induced arrhythmias during dialysis is often difficult to predict and depends upon the time of administration of digitalis, the amount of previous history of sensitivity, electrolyte balance, and rate of ion shifts, of which the latter is least available for analysis since membrane transport cannot be assessed. Not infrequently, digitalis arrhythmias are encountered after dialysis.

It has also been noted[28] that digitalized patients exhibit toxic manifestations during the first dialysis but rarely during subsequent dialyses, although the mechanism is unclear.

Changes in Serum Potassium and Calcium

Changes in serum K^+ in patients with chronic renal and heart disease are invariably observed. Elevated K^+ results in electrocardiographic changes and clinical signs and symptoms. Of the latter, confusion, muscular paralysis, and listlessness are the most prevalent. Morphologic changes in the electrocardiogram have been well described in both animals and humans. Peaking of the T waves occurs at serum K^+ levels of 5 to 8 mEq/L. At 7 to 9 mEq/L the ST segments become depressed, and the T wave may become biphasic. At serum K^+ levels of 8 to 9 mEq/L, atrial conduction defects become apparent and the P waves usually disappear at 10 to 11 mEq/L. Evidence for AV junctional and intraventricular conduction disturbances appears at serum K^+ of 10 mEq/L and more, leading to complete AV block and ventricular flutter and fibrillation at 14 to 16 mEq/L. In hyperkalemic toxicity, the most commonly observed arrhythmias are associated with disturbances of conduction. Hyperkalemia selectivity affects atrial muscle and probably accounts for loss of the P wave, although SA function persists. Altered conduction in the AV node results in first degree heart block and rarely Wenckebach AV conduction. This may progress to complete heart block or AV dissociation. As K^+ concentration rises, it depolarizes the myocardial cells leading to slow conduction which, in turn, facilitates reentrant arrhythmias. In addition, depolarization of cells may bring the resting membrane potential closer to threshold potential and increase cell excitability which is also arrhythmogenic.

Because of the association of lowering serum K^+ and the onset of digitalis induced arrhythmias, it might be expected that dialysis induced reduction in K^+ might precipitate arrhythmias. In Rubin's series,[29] 6 patients had regression of hyperkalemia during hemodialysis, none of whom developed arrhythmias. However, 11 of 33 patients did exhibit arrhythmias. These arrhythmias included ventricular premature beats, paroxysmal atrial beats, and junction rhythms (4 of the 5 latter rhythms in association with digitalis). Correction of both hypocalcemia and/or hyperkalemia resulted in transient arrhythmias and which ion, if any, was of primary importance could not be delineated. Although K^+ is such an important intracellular and extracellular ion, it is difficult to ascribe the arrhythmias during hyperkalemia or dialysis to this ion alone. Del Greco[30] has shown predialysis patients with hypokalemia who developed arrhythmias despite increasing serum K^+. Electrocardiographic and electrolyte studies suggested to these authors that a rise in plasma Ca^{++} may be more important for the induction of arrhythmias than the change in plasma K^+. However, there is little doubt that dialysis reduces serum and total body potassium. This reduction has well documented effects on automaticity and increases the slope of spontaneous depolarization. This leads to arrhythmias which are predominantly considered to be automatic and are clinically evident as nonparoxysmal junctional tachycardias and "slow ventricular tachycardias."

Magnesium

Knowledge about the role of magnesium in the heart has recently expanded and reports of hypomagnesemia[31,32] and associated arrhythmias are becoming more prevalent. Again, it is difficult to ascertain with certainty a specific cause for arrhythmias since several ion imbalances exist. Hypermagnesemia is found in renal failure and dialysis does reduce serum magnesium levels. It has been suggested[29,30] that a too rapid reduction in magnesium may precipitate ventricular arrhythmias. The appearance of ventricular extrasystolic beats and short runs of ventricular tachycardia may be secondary to hypomagnesemia and magnesium sulphate may be required.

Other Causes of Arrhythmias

Because of the questionable[3] high association of chronic renal failure with coronary artery disease, it is likely that any arrhythmias seen in coronary artery disease will be seen in chronic renal failure. Moreover, the ionic imbalances in renal failure may potentiate or exacerbate these arrhythmias. In addition, early rapid blood flow into the dialysis may result in the precipitation of angina and other cardiac arrhythmias. This problem is best handled by devices which reduce this initial load on the cardiovascular system.

Occasionally, arrhythmias during or after dialysis are encountered and no discernible cause appears evident. These arrhythmias are often transient but may be serious and result in death.[29] These arrhythmias maybe due to volume overload and cardiac chamber enlargement, but the precise mechanisms are undefined. In most cases, however, the arrhythmias are often supraventricular and terminate shortly after dialysis termination. It is plausible that some of these atrial tachyarrhythmias are associated with pericarditis and this diagnosis should be excluded by auscultatory and electrocardiographic means (Chapter 5).

Electrocardiographic Changes

Discussions of the electrocardiographic changes with dialysis have been reviewed elsewhere.[27,30] The electrolyte changes are predominant and overshadow a meaningful interpretation of ST and T abnormalities. No ion level has a specific electrocardiographic pattern but within certain ranges there are respective electrocardiographic manifestations for both Ca^{++}[33] and K^+.[34] Yet despite these some degree of superimposed "nonspecificity" must exist since so many other factors affect repolarization and are not in equilibrium during dialysis. Such changes in the ST and T waves are nonspecific and their meaning often cannot be gleaned even by the experienced electrocardiographer.

THERAPY OF ARRHYTHMIAS

A detailed description of antiarrhythmic agents in renal failure is discussed in detail elsewhere in Chapter 3. First, the arrhythmia must be recognized and, therefore, mandates that the patients at risk to develop arrhythmias should be monitored. The timing, appearance, type, and associated contributing factors must all be analyzed and weighed as to their importance and relationship to the observed arrhythmias. It would be of little value, for instance, to therapeutically pursue rapid transient atrial arrhythmias associated with hyperkalemia. Digitalis toxic arrhythmias, on the other hand, present a problem. Most of these arrhythmias are also transient but may occasionally persist. The clinician must, therefore, carefully assess the status of digitalization, and care must be taken to correct hypokalemia and hypercalcemia. Antiarrhythmic drugs are often not required if these ions are appropriately managed.

REFERENCES

1.   Mulligan, R.M.: Metastatic calcification. Arch. Path. 43:197, 1946.
2.   Terman, D.S., Alfrey, A.C., Hammond, W.S., et al.: Cardiac calcification in

uremia. A clinical biochemical and pathologic study. Am. J. Med. 50:744, 1971.

3. Nicholls, A.J., Catto, G.R.D., and Edward, N.: Accelerated atherosclerosis in long-term dialysis and renal transplant patterns. Fact or Fiction? Lancet 1:276, 1980.

4. Bulkey, B.H., Ridolfi, R.L., Salyer, W.R., et al.: Myocardial lesion of progressive systemic sclerosis. Circulation 53 (5):483, 1976.

5. Oram, S., and Stokes, W.: The heart in scleroderma. Br. Heart J. 23:243, 1961.

6. Escudero, J., and McDevitt, E.: The electrocardiogram in scleroderma: analysis of 60 cases and review of the literature. Am. Heart J. 56(6):846, 1958.

7. Thieme, G., Balente, M., and Rossi, L: Involvement of the cardiac conducting system in panarteritis nodosa. Am. Heart J. 95(6):716, 1978.

8. Leonhardt, E.J.G., Jacobson, H., and Rinqqvist, O.J.A.: Angiographic and clinicophysiologic investigation of a case of polyarteritis nodosa. Am J. Med 53:242, 1972.

9. Walts, A.E., and Dubois, E.L.: Acute dissecting aneurysm of the aorta as the fatal event in systemic lupus erythematosus. Am. Heart J. 93(3):387, 1977.

10. Wray, R., and Iveson, M.: Complete heart block and systemic lupus erythematosus. Br. Heart J. 37(9):982, 1972.

11. DelRio, A., Vazquez, J.J., Sobrino, J.A., et al.: Myocardial involvement in systemic lupus erythematosus. Chest 74(4):414, 1978.

12. Chew, C., Ziady, G.M., Raphael, M.J., et al.: The functional defect in amyloid heart disease. Am. J. Cardiol. 36:438, 1975.

13. Meaney, E., et al.: Cardiac amyloidosis, constrictive pericarditis and restrictive cardiomyopathy. Am. J. Cardiol. 38:547, 1976.

14. deFreitas, A.F., and Barbedo, A.: Conduction disturbances in 190 patients with familial amyloidotic polyneuropathy (Andrade's Type). Adv. Cardiol. 21:206, 1978.

15. Mehta, J., Tuna, N., Moller, J.H., et al.: Electrocardiographic and vectorcardiographic observations in Fabry's disease. Adv. Cardiol. 21:220, 1978.

16. Becker, A.E., Schoorl, R., Balk, A.G., et al.: Cardiac manifestations of Fabry's disease. Am. J. Cardiol. 36:829, 1975.

17. Khan, A.H., and Spodick, D.H.: Rheumatoid heart disease. Semin. Arthritis Rheum. 1:327, 1972.

18. Lebovitz, W.B.: The heart in rheumatoid arthritis (rheumatoid disease). Ann. Intern. Med. 58:102, 1963.

19. Lev, M., Bharati, S., Hoffman, F.G., et al.: The conduction system in rheumatoid arthritis with complete atrioventricular block. Am. Heart J. 90(1):78, 1975.

20. Ackerman, G.L., Doherty, J.E., and Flanigan, W.J.: Peritoneal dialysis and hemodialysis of tritiated digoxin. Ann. Intern. Med. 67:718, 1967.

21. Akera, T., and Brody, T.M.: Membrane adenosine triphosphatase: The effect of potassium on the formation and dissociation of ouabain-enzyme complex. J. Pharm. Exp. Ther. 166:545, 1971.

22. Murphy, R.B., Kidwai, A.M., and Daniel, E.E.: The uptake of cardiac glycosides by rabbit and rat myometrium. J. Pharm. Exp. Ther. 182:166, 1972.

23. Vassalle, M., Karis, J., and Hoffman, B.F.: Toxic effects of ouabain on Purkinje fibers and ventricular muscle fibers. Am. J. Physiol. 203:433, 1962.

24. Woodbury, L.A., and Hecht, H.H.: Effects of cardiac glycosides upon the electrical activity of single ventricular fibers of the frog heart and their relation to the digitalis effect of the electrocardiogram. Circulation 6:172, 1954.

25. Ferrier, G.R., and Moe, G.K.: Effect of calcium on acetylstrophanthidin-induced transient depolarizations in canine Purkinje tissue. Circ. Res. 33:508, 1973.

26. Ferrier, G.R., Saunders, J.H., and Mendez, C.: A cellular mechanism for the generation of ventricular arrhythmias by acetylstrophanthidin. Circ. Res. 32:600, 1973.

27. Castleman, L., Goldberg, M., Zuckerman, S., et al.: Selected electrocardiographic changes during acute renal failure and hemodialysis. Am. J. Cardiol. 12:841, 1963.

28. Merrill, J.P.: The use of the artificial kidney in the treatment of glomerulonephritis. J. Chron. Dis. 5:138, 1957.

29. Rubin, A.L., Lubash, G.D., Cohen, B.D., et al.: Electrocardiographic changes during hemodialysis with the artificial kidney. Circulation 18:227, 1958.

30. delGreco, F., and Grummer, H.: Electrolyte and electrocardiographic changes in the course of hemodialysis. Am. J. Cardiol. 9:43, 1962.

31. Singh, R.B., Singh, U.P., and Bajpai, H.S.: Refractory cardiac arrhythmias due to hypomagnesemia. ACTA Cardiologia 30:499, 1975.

32. Iseri, L.T., Freed, J., and Brues, A.R.: Magnesium deficiency and cardiac disorders. Am. J. Med. 88:837, 1975.

33. Yu, P.N.: The electrocardiographic changes associated with hypercalcemia and hypocalcemia. Am. J. Med. Sci. 224:413, 1952.

34. Winkler, A.W., Hoff, H.E., and Smith, P.K.: Electrocardiographic changes and concentrations of potassium in serum following intravenous injection of potassium chloride. Am. J. Physiol. 124:478, 1938.

9

HYPERTENSION THERAPY IN CHRONIC RENAL FAILURE

DAVID T. LOWENTHAL, M.D.

The treatment of hypertension, regardless of cause, must be based on a knowledge of the underlying pathohemodynamic state of the circulation (see Chapter 2). Amelioration of the intractable hypertension associated with intense vasoconstriction due to a vasopressor substance(s) previously required bilateral nephrectomy. Currently, dialysis and a pharmacologic approach, based on the availability of effective drugs and an understanding of their metabolism and kinetics in renal failure, provide a rational schema for the therapy of hypertension in the patient with end-stage renal disease.

PATHOHEMODYNAMICS OF HYPERTENSION

The hemodynamic changes in hypertensive patients with early nonuremic chronic renal parenchymal disease are quite similar to those that can be seen in the early stages of uncomplicated essential hypertension [1,2] Both groups of patients have an elevated cardiac output accompanied by an increase in heart rate. These factors are responsible for the increase in blood pressure, since total peripheral resistance is normal, and usually occur in patients who have mild renal insufficiency of less than 2 years' duration. The patient who has had renal insufficiency for longer than 2 years usually has a normal cardiac output and an increase in peripheral resistance. Similarly, with time, in the patient with untreated essential hypertension, an increase in peripheral resistance sustains the elevation of pressure.

Kim and coworkers[3] have extensively investigated the hypertension

155

associated with end-stage renal failure (see Chapter 2 for more detailed account). When the hemodynamics of advanced renal failure in dialysis patients are considered, regardless of blood pressure, and are compared with those of normal volunteers, the distinguishing features are anemia (mean hematocrit, 23 percent), increased heart rate and cardiac output, and normal total peripheral resistance. This hyperdynamic circulatory state is associated with an elevation in mean arterial pressure. Correction of the anemia with transfusions eliminates the hypoxic stimulus to "vasodilate" and, as a consequence, peripheral resistance and diastolic pressure rise.

Further analysis of uremia patients, divided into hypertensive and nonhypertensive groups, reveals that when hematocrit, cardiac output, heart rate, and stroke volume are comparable in the two groups, the mean arterial pressure elevation in the hypertensive uremic is maintained by a significant rise in total peripheral resistance.

When bilateral nephrectomy[3,4] was a common procedure for the treatment of intractable hypertension, the expected ultimate response was predicated upon whether the patient had malignant hypertension in association with chronic parenchymal renal disease (Fig. 1). When patients with similar exchangeable total body sodium levels were compared, the response to bilateral nephrectomy in the patient with non-malignant hypertension was a fall in mean arterial pressure and total peripheral resistance, with no change in cardiac output; in the patient with malignant hypertension, mean arterial pressure and peripheral resistance fell to normal and cardiac output, heretofore decreased, rose.

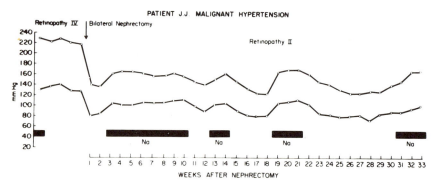

FIGURE 1. Clinical blood pressure response to bilateral nephrectomy. Patient's pressure is now dependent on salt and water balance. (With permission from Onesti, G.: Management and treatment of hypertension secondary to actue and chronic renal disease, *in* Genest, J. (ed): Hypertension: Pathophysiology and Treatment. McGraw-Hill, New York, 1977.)

Once nephrectomy is performed, some patients seem to be more sensitive to changes in salt and water balance.[5] In previously hypertensive anephric patients in whom bilateral nephrectomy is performed, blood pressure and peripheral resistance will increase when salt and water are infused. Thus, the patient who has previously been hypertensive does demonstrate some increased sensitivity to saline loading. On the other hand, patients who have bilateral nephrectomy in the setting of normotensive blood pressure (that is, pretransplantation for immunologic related or infection related parenchymal renal disease) do not necessarily have this response to salt and water. Therefore, patients can be divided into two groups, namely, those who are salt resistant and those who are salt sensitive. The proffered reasons for this response to saline loading in previously hypertensive anephric patients include the following: genetic predisposition; salt and water loading of the arteriolar wall is more conspicuous in previously challenged hypertensive arterioles; structural changes in the arterioles causing a decreased adaptability of the circulation to fluid expansion; and, finally, sympathetic activity is increased in hypertension, and this may be more prominent in postnephrectomy patients who were previously hypertensive.

There is no proof that the removal of the vasopressor component (contributed by diseased kidneys), which may have been responsible for the high mean arterial pressure, the high total peripheral resistance, and the subsequent increase in cardiac index, is mediated only by the renin-angiotensin system. In addition, there is no increased vascular sensitivity to endogenous or infused angiotensin in end-stage renal disease in the physiologically or anatomically anephric patient. The lack of a pressure response in previously normotensive anephric patients negates the previously conceived notion of renoprival hypertension (see Chapter 2).

TREATMENT OF HYPERTENSION

In early renal disease, hypertension is associated with an increase in peripheral vascular resistance with minimal, if any, increase in extracellular volume. As renal insufficiency progresses, the role of extracellular volume becomes more important. There is a close correlation between systolic blood pressure and extracellular volume or total body exchangeable sodium in patients with chronic renal failure (Fig. 2).[6] This relationship is even more direct in the anephric patient.[7] In concert with these mechanisms is the role of the renin-angiotensin-aldosterone system in terminal renal failure.[8] This chapter will concentrate on accepted therapeutic regimens which incorporate the principles of volume and vasoconstriction.

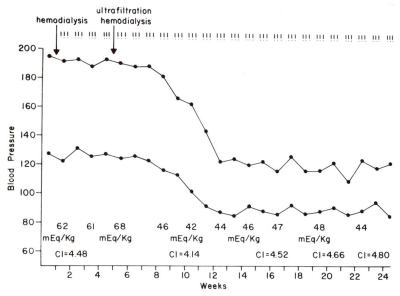

FIGURE 2. Removal of excess salt and water by ultrafiltration with resulting fall in blood pressure and increase in cardiac index. (With permission from Onesti, G.: Management and treatment of hypertension secondary to acute and chronic renal disease, *in* Genest, J. (ed): Hypertension: Pathophysiology and Treatment. McGraw-Hill, New York, 1977.)

The Role of Dialysis

The importance of extracellular volume expansion in the production of hypertension is demonstrated by the large number of hypertensive patients (70 to 75 percent) whose blood pressure can be controlled by means of sequential ultrafiltration or hemodiafiltration during hemodialysis or by peritoneal dialysis using hyperosmotic solutions.[6-14] (See Chapters 4 and 7). The removal of fluid by means of ultrafiltration or hemofiltration causes a reduction in the patient's weight, contraction of intravascular volume, and, thus, normalization of blood pressure without significant cardiovascular instability during the procedure. This reduced body weight, accompanied by normalization of blood pressure, is referred to as "dry weight."[12] Once dry weight is achieved and normal extracellular fluid volume is maintained, hypertensive eyeground changes may improve, the heart size may decrease, and improvement in the electrocardiogram may be seen.

Technically, ultrafiltration is accompanied by increased hydrostatic pressure within the blood compartment of the dialyzer, either by increasing resistance of venous return to the patient or by increasing the negative pressure on the dialysate side; both maneuvers increase the amount of fluid removed. Hemofiltration techniques will allow for the removal of fluid over a prolonged period (5 to 6 hours) and is hemodynamically well tolerated, but the removal of small molecular weight substances is much less than with hemodialysis. In those patients who are treated by means of peritoneal dialysis, hypertonic dialysis solutions are frequently utilized to remove excess sodium and water from the body. If hyponatremia is present as a result of expanded extracellular fluid volume, the hypertonic glucose solutions in the peritoneal fluid will cause an increase in serum sodium concentration, resulting from a proportionately greater removal of extracellular water than of sodium. This is not dependent on the development of hyperglycemia or on sodium diffusion from dialysate to extracellular fluid.[15,16]

These techniques will result in ultrafiltration rates of 12 to 18 ml/min or 3 to 6 kg of weight loss per treatment. The hemodialysis treatment must be performed three times per week in order to assure adequate control of hypertension; additional measures during dialysis to accomplish this goal may include using more frequent or longer dialysis periods, increasing the membrane surface area, selecting a more efficient dialyzer, and using bicarbonate in the dialysate all of which will aid in fluid removal and maintain vascular stability.[14]

If the dialysis approach, that is, ultrafiltration, is unsuccessful in the correction of the hypertension, then antihypertensive medications should be considered. These drugs may be used singly or in combination. If the patient has any degree of renal function, high doses of furosemide may be employed; in addition, the use of beta-blocking drugs, centrally acting antihypertensives and, lastly, vasodilators may be necessary in the treatment of the hypertension. If all of these measures fail, then bilateral nephrectomy may be considered.

Dialysis patients may require an alteration in dosage of antihypertensive drugs because the altered pharmacokinetics secondary to end-stage renal disease impair elimination (see Chapter 3). The following drugs may be employed adjunctively with dialysis in the treatment of hypertension in the dialysis patient.

Drug Therapy (Tables 1 and 2)

DIURETICS

When creatinine clearance is decreased to as low as 30 ml/min in the predialysis setting and as low as 2 ml/min in dialysis patients, furosemide

TABLE 1. Hemodynamic* and pharmacokinetic parameters of drugs used in chronic renal insufficiency

Drug Type	Cardiac Output (CO)	Total Peripheral Resistance (TPR)	Plasma Volume	Plasma Renin Activity	Half-Life in Renal Failure	Toxic Effects in Renal Disease
Diuretics						
Mild-moderate azotemia (i.e., creatinine clearance > 30 ml/min) Thiazides Chlorthalidone Metolazone	↓Acutely; then normal in 6–8 weeks	↓Chronically	↓	↑	No data	May convert asymptomatic hyperuricemia to overt gout
Moderate-severe azotemia (i.e., creatinine clearance < 30 ml/min) Furosemide	↓Acutely can↑ if heart failure is present	Acutely No data chronically	↓	↑	(?)Prolonged not dialyzable	Neurosensory ototoxicity can be permanent
Adrenergic inhibitors						
Propranolol	↓	↑	No change	↓	Unchanged to decreased; not dialyzable	May worsen renal failure because of negative inotropic action

Clonidine	(Not by negative inotropism)	Unchanged to ↓	Acutely↑ No change from control chronically	→	Prolonged; 50% of clonidine is excreted unchanged by kidney	Ultrafiltration may lead to postdialysis orthostatic response
Alpha-methyl-dopa	No change from control	↓	Acutely↑ No data chronically	→	Evidence suggests prolonged elimination phase; can be dialyzed	May have exaggerated response at equivalent dose given to normals
Prazosin	No change from control	↓	No change	→	Unchanged	First dose syncope; orthostatic hypotension
Vasodilators						
Minoxidil	↑	↓	↑	↑	No change from normals; probably dialyzable	Edema; T-wave inversion on ECG; pericardial effusion (?)
Hydralazine	↑	↓	↑	↑	Prolonged; plasma concentrations elevated	Angina

*Hemodynamic parameters are based on subjects with normal to mild renal insufficiency.

TABLE 2. Therapeutic regimen of drugs in
chronic renal failure

	Range of daily dose (begin with lowest dose and titrate to maximum)
Diuretic	
	Unlimited
Furosemide	80–1000 mg
Adrenergic inhibitors	
Metoprolol	50–200 mg
Propranolol	160–600 mg
Clonidine	0.2–1.2 mg
Alpha-methyldopa	1.0–2.0 gm
Prazosin	1–20 mg
Vasodilators	
Minoxidil	10–80 mg
Hydralazine	50–200 mg

is still effective and essentially has no dose limitation (200 to 2000 mg). Although furosemide enhances urine formation, natriuresis, kaliuresis, and urea excretion, it is not a substitute for maintenance dialysis. It may, however, allow a synergistic and flexible regimen for fluid and electrolyte balance and blood pressure control.

Initially, when furosemide is given parenterally, there is an acute fall in cardiac output, but cardiac output can increase if heart failure is present. The increase is attributed to two mechanisms: an increase in compliance in the pulmonary circulation and peripheral venous pooling. Of special significance is the fact that in renal failure, the biologic elimination half-life of furosemide is prolonged.[17] It is not a dialyzable moiety, and, in addition, neurosensory ototoxicity is always a possibility, although there are few reported instances of this complication. On the other hand, the incidence of neurosensory ototoxicity is significant with ethacrynic acid and increases as renal insufficiency worsens. Furosemide also may cause some nephrotoxicity related to its metabolic conversion to a metabolite that can become convalenty bound to tissue macromolecules and act as an alkylating agent, causing tissue necrosis.[18] One should not attempt to give "megadoses" of furosemide, e.g., 1000 to 2000 mg/day.[19,20] If renal function is so compromised, it pays to "Be wise and dialyze."

Adrenergic Inhibitors

BETA-ADRENERGIC BLOCKADE

Only propranolol will be discussed here because of the large experience in ESRD. The half-life of propranolol in renal disease is either unchanged or decreased.[21] It is not dialyzable, and it is tightly protein bound.[22] Renal failure may worsen in patients on propranolol, because of its negative inotropic effect which in sequence may result in a fall in GRF and renal blood flow.[23] The acute and multiple dose pharmacokinetics of propranolol in chronic renal insufficiency are discussed in detail in Chapter 3. Briefly, in normal patients given 80 mg of propranolol, the elimination half-life is approximately 4 hours. On the other hand, in patients with chronic renal insufficiency studied on an interdialysis day, the plasma concentration is significantly elevated (mean, 154 ng/ml), peaking at about 90 min. The elimination half-life is slightly less (3.3 hours), yet statistically not different from that in the normal controls. When given by mouth at doses of 30 mg or less, propranolol is extensively metabolized by the liver, so that very little remains to provide pharmacologic activity.[24] From mathematical analyses, it was inferred that the liver metabolizes propranolol abnormally at an 80 mg dose, yielding more drug to the circulation for pharmacologic activity. It was concluded that the first-pass effect of propranolol is altered in patients with renal disease,[21] but that a contracted volume of distribution may coexist.

A comparison between patients with renal insufficiency who were given 80 mg of propranolol acutely and patients who received 40 to 80 mg of propranolol chronically produced results suggesting a short biologic half-life in the latter group.[22,25] Similarly, other drugs that have been studied, such as diphenylhydantoin,[26] guanethidine,[27] and antipyrine[28] all have an accelerated rate of metabolism in renal disease. Despite this enhanced rate of metabolism, accumulation of the 4-OH propranolol metabolite may provide the antihypertensive effect observed in patients.

When indicated the combination of propranolol with diuretic or dialysis and vasodilator has proven to be an effective and standard form of therapy.

CENTRALLY ACTING ANTIHYPERTENSIVES

Clonidine[29,30]

It is safe to give this drug in customary doses (0.2 to 1.2 mg daily) to patients with renal insufficiency despite the fact that the elimination half-life is prolonged as azotemia progresses. The hepatic metabolism of the drug accounts for 50 percent of clonidine elimination and the kidney accounts for the elimination of the other 50 percent of clonidine and its metabolites (activity?). Theoretically an increase or poor blood pressure response may indicate a plasma concentration of clonidine in excess of 2 ng per ml. This would cause stimulation of *peripheral* alpha receptors leading to vasoconstriction. Then a reduction in dosage would be necessary. We have observed plasma concentrations which are ten times greater with no adverse blood pressure response.

Clonidine suppresses plasma renin activity and, ultimately, the activity of angiotensin II, a known vasoconstricting or vasopressor component of hypertension. Therefore, when indicated clonidine, with diuretic or dialysis or with vasodilator, is an accepted and standard combination in the hypertensive armamentarium of ESRD.

Methyldopa

This is not the sympatholytic of choice when a potent vasodilator is to be given simultaneously—simply because it is not as effective in reducing the heart rate as either propranolol or clonidine. It is effective in mild to moderate hypertension at dosages up to 2000 mg daily, especially when combined with furosemide or dialysis or both. Evidence suggests that, in the anephric patient, the biologic elimination half-life is prolonged, and its accumulation may cause some increase in sensitivity to its hypotensive effects.[31] Methyldopa can be dialyzed.[32]

To date, it is not known whether there is refractoriness or tolerance after a period of time to the action of methyldopa or to the action of alpha-methylnorepinephrine, despite the fact that there are higher than normal plasma concentrations. It is clear, however, that the drug is not effective in *severe hypertension associated with end-stage renal disease.*

ALPHA-ADRENERGIC BLOCKADE

Prazosin[33-35]

This atypical alpha-adrenergic blocking drug is effective in a 3 to 8 mg dose range when given with diuretics to patients with hypertension, regardless of status of renal function. At higher doses, 9 to 20 mg per day, the action of prazosin may be blunted after prolonged use and because of the severity of the hypertension. Its action is then enhanced by adding clonidine or beta-blockade. Its elimination is unimpaired in ESRD.

ANGIOTENSIN II INHIBITION AND CONVERTING ENZYME INHIBITOR

A proportion of patients with chronic renal failure undergoing regular hemodialysis remains hypertensive despite sodium depletion.[36] In these, renin secretion from the diseased kidneys seems to be disproportionately stimulated and thus plasma angiotensin II is excessively high in relation to exchangeable sodium.[37-39] Bilateral nephrectomy can be strikingly effective,[36,40,41] but carries the disadvantage that erythropoietin, as well as renin, is reduced, and anemia may be worsened. Suppression of renin output by propranolol administration can be an alternative.[41,43] To test the renin axis, saralasin can be given acutely.[39] Captopril treatment is obviously rational, and seems a promising approach to this difficult problem.[44] The ability of captopril to reduce blood pressure in hypertensive patients with some renal impairment but not severe enough to require dialysis has been taken as suggestive evidence that these subjects may also have a disproportionate elevation of angiotensin II in relation to exchangeable sodium.[45]

VASODILATORS

The vasodilator drugs play an important role in the pharmacologic management of the hypertensive patient with renal disease. Minoxidil is effective in the dialysis patient whose diastolic blood pressure exceeds 120 mm Hg; hydralazine is useful in renal insufficiency associated with mild to moderate hypertension, that is, diastolic blood pressures of 105 to 120 mm Hg.

Minoxidil

The onset of action of minoxidil is rapid and occurs within 1 to 2 hours after oral administration of 5 to 10 mg. The pharmacologic effect of the drug differs from that predicted by the biologic half-life. Minoxidil is extensively metabolized by hepatic oxidation and glucuronide conjugation. The biologic half-life is relatively short (about 4 hours) in patients with normal renal function and in those with chronic renal disease; there appears to be no significant accumulation of the drug in patients with impaired renal function.[46,47] Despite the rapid elimination of minoxidil from the circulation, the pharmacologic effect of the drug can last more than 12 hours. Patients who are given one dose of minoxidil a day are still under optimum control 24 hours later. The bioavailability is significant, even though there is only a small amount in the circulation, because the drug is only minimally protein bound, and more free drug is bound to tissue.

A significant antihypertensive effect is seen within 48 to 72 hours.[48] The pretreatment mean arterial pressure in a group of azotemic patients was approximately 160 mm Hg. Within 72 hours after a mean dose of 13.5 mg, there was a fall in mean arterial pressure to approximately 106 mm Hg. After 1 year of treatment, mean arterial pressure was stabilized at around 100 mm Hg. The patients tolerated the acute reduction in mean arterial pressure and, with concurrent therapy, that is, a diuretic or dialysis and a bradycardic drug such as propranolol or clonidine, they were able to maintain normotensive levels and to avoid bilateral nephrectomy. Maintaining the diseased kidneys in situ has some advantages; there may still be some erythropoietin stimulating effect maintaining hematopoiesis, which obviates the need for additional transfusions, as well as some ability of the kidneys to convert 25-hydroxycholecalciferol to the active 1,25-dihyroxycholecalciferol necessary for calcium phosphorus-bone homeostasis.

Minoxidil, like other vasodilators, also causes an increase in peripheral renin activity (Table 3). Minoxidil may be able to override the renin suppressing effect of propranolol at the juxtaglomerular apparatus, but it cannot override the effect of propranolol on the heart when the plasma propranolol concentration is within therapeutic range, that is, 50 to 100 ng/ml.[48,49]

As a vasodilator, minoxidil causes significant plasma volume expansion with consequent sodium and water retention. Furosemide may be given to achieve adequate volume contraction. For those who no longer have adequate renal function to respond to a diuretic, hemodialysis or peritoneal dialysis may be necessary.

Early electrocardiographic changes, that is, reversible ischemic T wave inversion, may occur in approximately 25 percent of patients receiving minoxidil. Vasodilator induced tachycardia is kept under control with either propranolol or clonidine. Hirsutism, the mechanisms for which are

TABLE 3. Examples of plasma renin activity (PRA) (ng/ml $\times$ hr) and heart rate (HR) before treatment with propranolol (P) and with propranolol and minoxidil (M)

	Control		P		P & M	
	PRA	HR	PRA	HR	PRA	HR
1.	11.4	80	1.2	56	3.4	60
2.	5.0	82	1.9	68	4.7	68
3.	0.26	86	0.3	76	0.74	74

nebulous, can be managed with depilatory agents. Pericardial effusion has been reported with minoxidil in patients on dialysis. It is difficult to discern whether this is part of the natural course of end-stage renal disease or due to minoxidil. Echocardiograms taken sequentially from 12 patients over a 2 year period reveal no evidence of pericardial effusion.[51]

Hydralazine

Hydralazine is a less potent vasodilator drug; in fact, there is virtually no comparison with minoxidil, particularly in severe hypertension with end-stage renal insufficiency. The plasma levels of hydralazine accumulate, and the half-life of the drug may be prolonged.[50,52] The acetylation phenotype of patients may contribute to this prolonged elimination as well as to the hydralazine induced lupus syndrome. Side effects are similar to those of minoxidil except for the absence of hirsutism. Hydralazine can cause fluid retention and, in addition, can cause significant coronary artery ischemia, resulting in angina pectoris. Because of these effects, propranolol and clonidine are the drugs of choice for the control of heart rate, and furosemide or dialysis or both for control of salt and water balance.

OTHER AGENTS

Guanethidine has a rapid rate of metabolism in renal failure,[27] yet pharmacodynamically, the propensity to orthostatic hypotension in addition to ultrafiltration from dialysis makes this drug contraindicated in the dialysis patient with severe hypertension.

The Role of Bilateral Nephrectomy

Despite the use of ultrafiltration dialysis and maximum doses of antihypertensive medications, there is a small number of dialysis patients in whom hypertension may not be correctable. Such patients have been shown to respond to bilateral nephrectomy, particularly when the hypertension is associated with elevated peripheral renin levels.[15] Hemodynamically, this situation is associated with a marked increase in total peripheral resistance that is due to the increased activity of some vasopressor, probably the renin-angiotensin system.[5] In addition, if these patients have malignant hypertension, cardiac index will increase after bilateral nephrectomy.[3] After the bilateral nephrectomy and resolution of the hypertension, detectable renin levels are very low or absent.[53] The major objections and disadvantages to bilateral nephrectomy are decreased erythropoietic activity—resulting in lower hematocrit, increased transfusion requirements[54] and the absence of renal mass—which, when present, had produced 1,25-dihydroxycholecalciferol, the most active form of vitamin D.[55] It must be considered that the malignant or refractory hypertension is of far greater consequence to the patient than is the increase in transfusion requirements and the possible worsening of osteodystrophy. This, in effect, justifies the bilateral nephrectomy procedure in the treatment of refractory hypertension.

CONCLUSION

Hypertension in dialysis patients is usually related to an excess of extracellular fluid volume (see Fig. 2). In 70 to 75 percent of cases, ultrafiltration by peritoneal or hemodialysis will restore blood pressure to normal. The remaining patients have hypertension that may not be correctable by ultrafiltration. The hypertension is usually a result of an increase in total peripheral resistance in class and characteristically responds to drugs that have centrally acting antihypertensive properties, e.g., clonidine, methyldopa, prazosin, beta-blockers, and vasodilators. Peripheral sympathetic inhibitors impair the ability of the cardiovascular system to adjust to the rapid changes in blood volume. Thus, guanethidine and reserpine should not be used in these patients. If these agents do not effect a reduction in blood pressure then bilateral nephrectomy may be considered; a small number of patients may respond with normalization of blood pressure attendent to the removal of a vasopressor substance(s) which may be related to overactivity of the renin-angiotensin system (see Fig. 2).

Hemodialysis patients needing bilateral nephrectomy for the control of hypertension include: 1) maintenance hemodialysis patients with hypertension resistant to ultrafiltration dialysis, salt and water restriction, and appropriate drug therapy; 2) most patients with malignant hypertension, severe weight loss, and persistant clinical deterioration; 3) hypertensive patients who cannot tolerate antihypertensive drugs. Clinically, the blood pressure after bilateral nephrectomy becomes easier to control with ultrafiltration dialysis and drug therapy.

The principles of drug administration and the selection of drugs in the anephric state are the same as in the maintenance hemodialysis patients before bilateral nephrectomy. Despite the consideration that the renin suppressive effect of methyldopa and clonidine may contribute to the antihypertensive efficacy of these drugs, both methyldopa and clonidine lower the blood pressure effectively in anephric humans (Table 4).

TABLE 4. Choice of antihypertensive agents and management

	In Patients on Hemodialysis
Step I	Dietary salt restriction and ultrafiltration dialysis
Step II	Methyldopa
	Clonidine
	Beta-blocker with prazosin
	Contraindicated: guanethidine
Step III	Hydralazine (with methyldopa or clonidine)
	Prazosin (with methyldopa)
Step IV	Beta-blocker with minoxidil
Step V	If blood pressure not normalized or side effects of medications intolerable, bilateral nephrectomy

REFERENCES

1. Onesti, G., Kim, K.E., Fernandes, M., et al.: Hypertension of renal parenchymal disease, in Giovanetti, S., Bonomini, V., D'Amico, G. (eds.): Proceedings of the Sixth International Congress of Nephrology, Florence 1975. S. Karger, Basel, 1976, p. 284.

2. Lund-Johansen, P.: Hemodynamic alterations in essential hypertension, in Onesti, G., Kim, K.E., Moyer, J.H. (eds.): Hypertension: Mechanisms and Management. Grune & Stratton, New York, 1973, p. 43.

3. Kim, K.E., Onesti, G., Schwartz, A., et al.: Hemodynamics of hypertension in chronic end-stage renal disease. Circulation 46:456, 1972.

4. Briggs, W.A., Light, J., Yeager, H., et al.: Nephrectomy in selected patients with severe refractory hypertension receiving dialysis. Surg. Gynecol. Obstet. 141:251, 1975.

5. Onesti, G., Kim, K.E., Greco, J.A., et al.: Blood pressure regulation in end-stage renal disease and anephric man. Circ. Res. 26(Suppl. I):145, 1975.

6. Wilkinson, R., Scott, D.F., Uldall, P.R., et al.: Plasma renin and exchangeable sodium in the hypertension of chronic renal failure. The effect of bilateral nephrectomy. Q. J. Med. (new series) 39(155):377, 1970.

7. Onesti, G., Swartz, C., Ramirez, O., et al.: Bilateral nephrectomy for control of hypertension in uremia. Trans. Am. Soc. Artif. Intern. Organs 14:361, 1968.

8. Weidmann, P., and Maxwell, M.H.: The renin-angiotensin-aldosterone system in terminal renal failure. Kidney Inter. 8:S219, 1975.

9. Miller, R.B., and Tassistro, C.R.: Peritoneal dialysis. N. Engl. J. Med. 281:945, 1969.

10. Hampl, H., Paeprer, H., Unger, V., et al.: Hemodynamics during hemodialysis sequential ultrafiltration and hemofiltration. J. Dialysis 3:51, 1979.

11. Henderson, L.W., Besarab, A., and Michaels, A.: Blood purification by ultrafiltration and fluid replacement (diafiltration). Trans. Am. Soc. Artif. Intern. Organs 13:216, 1967.

12. Ing, T.S., Ashback, D.L., Kanter, A., et al.: Fluid removal with negative-

pressure hydrostatic ultrafiltration using a partial vacuum. Nephron 14:451, 1975.

13. Shinaberger, J.H., Brantbar, N., Miller, J.H., et al.: Successful application of sequential hemofiltration followed by diffusion dialysis with standard dialysis equipment. Trans. Am. Soc. Artif. Intern. Organs 24:677, 1978.

14. Graefe, U., Milutinovich, J., Foltette, W.C., et al.: Less dialysis-induced morbidity and vascular instability with bicarbonate in dialysate. Ann. Intern. Med. 88:332, 1978.

15. Vertes, V., Cangiano, J.L., Berman, L.B., et al.: Hypertension in end-stage renal disease. N. Engl. J. Med. 280:978, 1969.

16. Nolph, K.D., Hano, J.E., and Teschan, P.E.: Peritoneal sodium transport during hypertonic peritoneal dialysis. Ann. Intern. Med. 70:931, 1969.

17. Cutler, R.E., Forrey, A.W., Christopher, T.G., et al.: Pharmacokinetics of furosemide in normal subjects and functionally anephric patients. Clin. Pharmacol. Ther. 15:588, 1974.

18. Mitchell, J.R., and Jollows, D.T.: Progress in hepatology: metabolic activation of drugs to toxic subjects. Gastroenterology 68(2):392, 1975.

19. Editorial: Big dose of furosemide in renal failure. Lancet 2:803, 1971.

20. Muth, R.G.: Diuretic properties of furosemide in renal disease. Ann. Intern. Med. 69:249, 1968.

21. Lowenthal, D.T., Briggs, W.A., Gibson, T.P., et al.: Pharmacokinetics of oral propranolol in chronic renal disease. Clin. Pharmacol. Ther. 16:761, 1974.

22. Lowenthal, D.T., and Mutterperl, R.E.: Steady-state propranolol half-life in chronic renal disease. Clin. Pharmacol. Ther. 19:111, 1976.

23. Bauer, J.H., and Brooks, C.S.: The long-term effect of propranolol therapy on renal function. Am. J. Med. 66:405, 1979.

24. Shand, D.G., and Rangno, R.E.: The disposition of propranolol. I. Elimination during oral absorption in man. Pharmacology 7:159, 1972.

25. Lowenthal, D.T.: Pharmacokinetics of propranolol, quinidine, procaine amide and lidocaine in chronic renal disease. Am. J. Med. 62:632, 1977.

26. Reidenberg, M.M., Odar-Cederlof, I., von Behr, C., et al.: Protein binding of diphenylhydantoin and desmethylimipramine in plasma from patients with poor renal function. N. Engl. J. Med. 285:264, 1971.

27. Rahn, K.H.: The influence of renal function on plasma levels, urinary excretion, metabolism and antihypertensive effect of guanethidine (Ismelin) in man. Clin. Nephrol. 1:14, 1973.

28. Lichter, M., Black, M., and Arias, I.M.: The metabolism of antipyrine in patients with chronic renal failure. J. Pharmacol. Exp. Ther. 187:612, 1973.

29. Wing, L.M.H., Reid, J.L., Davies, D.S., et al.: Pharmacokinetic and concentration effect relationships of clonidine in essential hypertension. Eur. J. Clin. Pharmacol. 12:463, 1977.

30. Hutler, H.N., Licht, J.H., Ilnick, L.P., et al.: Clinical efficacy and pharmacokinetics of clonidine in hemodialysis and renal insufficiency. J. Lab. Clin. Med. 94:223, 1979.

31. Myhre, E., Broadwall, E.K., Stenbaek, O., et al.: Plasma turnover of methyldopa in advanced renal failure. Acta Med. Scand. 191:343, 1972.

32. Yeh, B.K., Dayton, P.G., and Waters, W.C.: Removal of alpha-methyldopa in man by dialysis. Proc. Soc. Exp. Biol. Med. 135:840, 1970.

33. Lowenthal, D.T., Hobbs, D., Affrime, M.B., et al.: Prazosin kinetics and effectiveness in renal failure. Clin. Pharmacol. Ther. 27:779, 1980.

34. Lowenthal, D.T.: Clinical pharmacology of vasodilators. N.Y. State J. Med. 79:66, 1979.

35. Martinez, E.W., Fernandes, M., Fiorentini, R., et al.: Effectiveness of the combination prazosin-propranolol-diuretic in refractory hypertension. Clin. Pharmacol. Ther. 23:20, 1978.

36. Brown, J.J., Curtis, J.R., Lever, A.F., et al.: Plasma renin concentration and the control of blood pressure in patients on maintenance hemodialysis. Nephron 6:329, 1969.

37. Davies, D.L., Schalekamp, M.A., Beevers, D.G., et al.: Abnormal relation between exchangeable sodium and the renin-angiotensin system in malignant hypertension and in hypertension with chronic renal failure. Lancet 1:683, 1973.

38. Schalekamp, M.A., Beevers, D.G., Briggs, J.D., et al.: Hypertension in chronic renal failure: An abnormal relation between sodium and the renin-angiotensin system. Am. J. Med. 55:379, 1973.

39. Faden, S.Z. and Lifschitz, M.D.: Use of Saralasin in end-stage renal disease. Kidney Inter. 15:S93, 1979.

40. Brown, J.J., Dusterdieck, G., Fraser, R., et al.: Hypertension and chronic renal failure. Br. Med. Bull. 14:361, 1971.

41. Onesti, G., Swartz, C., Ramirez, O., et al.: Bilateral nephrectomy for control of hypertension in uremia. Trans. Am. Soc. Artif. Intern. Organs 14:361, 1968.

42. Maggiore, Q., Biagini, M., Zoccali, C., et al.: Long-term propranolol treatment of resistant arterial hypertension in hemodialysis patients. Clin. Sci. Mol. Med. 48(Suppl. 2):73, 1975.

43. Moore, S.B., and Goodwin, F.J.: Effect of beta-adrenergic blockade on plasma renin activity and intractable hypertension in patients receiving regular dialysis treatment. Lancet 2:67, 1976.

44. Vaughan, E.D., Carey, R.M., Ayers, C.R., et al.: Hemodialysis-resistant hypertension: control with an orally-active inhibitor of converting enzyme. J. Clin. Endocrinol. Metab. 48:869, 1979.

45. Brunner, H.R., Waeber, B., Wauters, J.P., et al.: Inappropriate renin secretion unmasked by captopril (SQ 14 225) in hypertension of chronic renal failure. Lancet 2:704, 1978.

46. Gottlieb, T.B., Thomas, R.C., and Chidsey, C.A.: Pharmacokinetic studies of minoxidil. Clin. Pharmacol. Ther. 13:436. 1972.

47. Lowenthal, D.T., Onesti, G., Mutterperl, R., et al.: Long-term clinical effects, bioavailability and kinetics of minoxidil in relation to renal function. J. Clin. Pharmacol. 18:500, 1978.

48. Mutterperl, R.E., Diamond, F.B., and Lowenthal, D.T.: Long-term effects of minoxidil in the treatment of malignant hypertension in chronic renal failure. J. Clin. Pharmacol. 16:498, 1976.

49. Velasco, M., O'Malley, K., Robin, N.W., et al.: Differential effects of propranolol on heart rate and plasma renin activity in patients treated with minoxidil. Clin. Pharmacol. Ther. 16:1031, 1974.

51. Lowenthal, D.T., and Kotler, M.: Unpublished observations.

50. Reidenberg, M.M., Drayer, D., DeMarco, A.L., et al.: Hydralazine elimination in man. Clin. Pharmacol. Ther. 14:970, 1973.

52. Lowenthal, D.T., Affrime, M.B., Onesti, G., et al.: Pharmacokinetics and effectiveness of antihypertensive vasodilators in chronic renal failure. Clin. Res. 26:291A, 1978.

53. Berman, L.B., Vertes, V., Mitra, S., et al.: Renin-angiotensin system in anephric patients. N. Engl. J. Med. 286:58, 1972.

54. Kominami, N., Lowrie, E.G., Ianhez, I.E., et al.: The effect of total nephrec-

tomy on hematopoiesis in patients undergoing chronic hemodialysis. J. Lab. Clin. Med. 78:524, 1971.

55.   Brickman, A.S., Coburn, J.W., and Norman, A.W.: Action of 1,25-dihydroxy-cholecalciferol, a potent kidney-produced metabolite of vitamin D_3 in uremic man. N. Engl. J. Med. 287:891, 1972.

10

MANAGEMENT OF INFECTIVE ENDOCARDITIS IN CHRONIC RENAL FAILURE

ANDREW R. SCHWARTZ, M.D. AND
CLIFFORD WLODAVER, M.D.

The definition of infective endocarditis has seemed relatively simple in the past. The presence of anemia, fever, a new or changing murmur coupled with embolic tissue, and multiple positive blood cultures has always seemed quite sufficient to the clinician to demonstrate endovascular infection. Corollary issues such as pre-existent endovascular prostheses, drug addiction, congenital or acquired degenerative valvular disease, and, more recently, parenteral drug abuse and cardiovascular surgical advances have added further dimensions to the predisposing factors involved in acquiring infection within the endocardial tissues.

In the last decade, an additional class of patients has entered the medical care system who present special problems of endovascular infection. These are the individuals with chronic renal insufficiency.[1] In this setting, patients with and without endogenous cardiac disease are given one of a variety of arteriovenous fistulous connections in order to prepare them for on-going hemodialysis. A smaller group of individuals is maintained on chronic peritoneal dialysis therapy. A few individuals in both groups after variable intervals of dialysis will progress to renal transplantation with their original arteriovenous accesses left intact for maintenance and emergency therapy. It is in this clinical setting that our definition of infective endocarditis must be broadened to include the endovascular foci of infection that are predisposed to and inherent in on-going dialytic therapy.

MICROBIOLOGY

Once an access site is placed in an extremity for dialytic therapy, opportunities occur two to three times weekly with each dialysis for contaminants (microorganisms) to enter the blood stream. The major concept in the accessibility of microorganisms to the blood stream of patients in on-going dialysis is the vulnerability of the access site to microbes. Most commonly, endogenous skin flora, including staphylococci—both S. aureus and S. epidermidis, micrococci, and enterococci and other streptococci, can be carried from the skin into the blood stream. In individuals suffering from renal insufficiency and mild acidosis, a phenomenon occurs with increasing gram-negative rod colonization of the skin with enteric gram-negatives such as Proteus, E. coli, and Klebsiella. Among those who spend increasing intervals in the hospital, other nosocomially acquired organisms such as Serratia and Pseudomonas may also become a problem due to skin colonization and potentially gain entry into the blood stream. Bacteria might be accidently applied to the skin puncture site through contaminated chemical soaps or other agents. If these cleansing solutions are contaminated or if the dialytic fluid itself is contaminated or if the equipment provides microbial access to the dialysate stream which then flows back into the patient, then an obvious portal of entry for systemic infection is present.

On occasion, a puncture site or skin focus near the area of arteriovenous access may be contaminated, and exuding microorganisms may then progress along the skin surface and even via the needle-skin access interface to enter the blood stream. Although the frequency of occurence of such invasions is low, its significance is still great to the patient with chronic renal insufficiency. Also, infections involving the urinary tract, respiratory tract, hollow viscera such as the bowel or gallbladder, or distant skin foci are examples of areas from which microorganisms may gain entry into the blood stream. A novel problem in this regard is the possibility of transmission of certain pathogens within the dialysis unit that, because of the proximity of individuals during dialysis therapy, may lead to endemic/epidemic spread within a particular dialysis unit, for example, the development of Salmonella gastroenteritis with ensuing bacteremia in a few patients and its dissemination throughout a dialysis unit. Fortunately, most individuals throughout their lifetime have recurrent bouts of bacteremia which are quite capably resolved by normal body defenses.

In the case of individuals who have increased turbulence or other areas of diminished host resistance within the endovascular structures, a process of local endovascular infection may result. This is analagous to infective endocarditis involving the endomural surface of the heart or heart valves, endarteritis or venous channel infection involving one of the other major blood vessels, or infection at an arteriovenous access site or fistula created for the purpose of chronic renal maintenance therapy by dialysis. Brief intradialytic and postdialytic episodes of fever are often due to either endotoxin or transient bacteremia associated with local colonization at the AV access site. Intermittent serous drainage from these venipuncture sites following dialysis, local colonization, and transient local foci of infection is also a common phenomenon. Nonetheless, most hosts on chronic renal dialysis therapy satisfactorily resolve these without developing symptomatic infection.

Unfortunately, bacteremic infection among individuals on hemodialysis is not at all unique. A recent article by Nsouli and associates[1] has pointed out that in their series of patients, 9.5 percent of patients on chronic hemodialysis had bacteremic infection and almost 11 percent with acute renal failure who were dialyzed had bacteremic infections. Staphylococcus aureus is overwhelmingly the most frequently isolated organism in all series of patients and in our own personal experience. This is to be expected in 50 to 60 percent of the bacteremic episodes among individuals on hemodialysis. The second most common microorganism involved is Staphylococcus epidermidis and this particular organism poses some special problems in interpretation. Clearly, it is very often encountered in blood cultures in most hospital laboratories, and because of its lack of coagulase it is frequently interpreted as a skin pathogen that is usually not significant and as a contaminant of the blood culture drawing process. Unfortunately, among those with prosthetic devices or artifical vessels or recurrent skin punctures, including those on hemodialysis, the presence of recurrently positive blood cultures for Staphylococcus epidermidis may indeed have pathologic significance. The net result is that although this is the second most commonly identified microorganism, it requires recurrent isolation in order to be interpreted as important in the individual's clinical course. After these two gram-positive cocci, the most common microorganisms in diminishing order are: negative rods including E. coli, Pseudomonas aeruginosa, Klebsiella pneumoniae, and Enterobacteriaceal, and gram-positive cocci, in particular the enterococcus, Streptococcus pneumoniae, and other streptococcal species.

Noteworthy is the fact that frequently these patients have more than one organism present in the blood at the same time. Combinations of staphylococci coagulase positive and negative rods, especially the Enterobacteriaceae, are the most frequently encountered combination. Fortunately, these microorganisms are present in a minority of hemodialysis patients with bacteremia, but the prevalence is greater than among other groups of bacteremic patients encountered in the hospital setting.

The incidence of microorganisms causing infective endocarditis in patients on hemodialysis is led overwhelmingly by Staphylococcus aureus followed by S. epidermidis, Pseudomonas aeruginosa, other gram-negative bacilli, members of the tribe Klebsiella, streptococci including enterococcus, diphtheroids, and Listeria monocytogenes.[2] Clearly, an excess of 60 percent of the patients with infective endocarditis were suffering from *Staphylococcus aureus* infection and more than three-quarters were suffering from gram-positive coccal infection. These latter facts are important in the empiric initiation of antimicrobial chemotherapy until the results of blood cultures and susceptibility testing can be obtained. Although bacteremia is a common phenomenon in the dialysis population, the actual incidence of infective endocarditis is estimated in several studies cited by Cross and Steigbigel at between 2.7 and 6.6 percent.[3-5]

The sites of infective endocarditis among hemodialysis patients are most commonly the valvular surfaces of the left side of the heart: the aortic valve being the most prominent, the mitral valve next, the tricuspid valve third, and the pulmonic fourth. Of great interest is the fact that most of the valvular infections occurred among individuals who did not have pre-existing valvular heart disease. Univalvular infection is far more common than multiple valvular infection among these patients as well.

The diagnosis of infective endocarditis becomes more of a challenge to the clinician in this population. The presence of fever, anemia, and murmur as independent phenomena is quite frequently noted among patients undergoing hemodialysis. Hematuria, if encountered in the limited urinary flow of some of these patients, has multiple explanations as does the presence of neurologic complications and metastatic sites of infection outside the cardiovascular system.

The usual criteria for the diagnosis of infective endocarditis include predisposing cardiac lesion, cardiac murmur—especially a changing one, fever, positive blood cultures, embolic issue, and, of course, the classic signs such as Janeway lesion, Osler's nodes, and petechial lesions. In the presence of these factors, the diagnosis of infective endocarditis becomes a relatively simple clinical decision. In the chronic renal insufficiency, febrile episodes associated with dialysis and extravascular sites as well as access sites of infection are relatively common phenomena. In renal failure, however, the patient might have only minimal changes in body temperature even though constitutional symptoms may be present at all times. Anemia is an ever present phenomenon among those with chronic renal failure, and so it becomes less significant in the differential diagnosis of infective endocarditis. Nonetheless, a marked change in the anemia from previous stable levels might be a useful sign to be considered. Bacteremia that can be documented by blood culture obviously should always raise the question of intravascular foci of infection. Nonetheless, as mentioned previously, the most common sources of bacteremia are access site infections, but transient bacteremia is usually the rule, and the seeding of viscera and the endocardial surface is a relatively uncommon phenomenon. Clearly then, it would require multiple positive blood cultures or some other phenomenon to increase the index of suspicion for the presence of endovascular or endocardial infection.

This might be provided by the development of a new murmur, especially where increasing cardiac failure might not be described or some other etiology for high output state can be ruled out. The presence of valvular insufficiency or evidence of unequivocal valvular dysfunction where none had previously existed in the face of adequate fluid and electrolyte balance might certainly be helpful. Should embolic issue, such as Janeway lesions, Osler's nodes, or petechial lesions be clearly demonstrated, again, the index for suspicion should be heightened. Concomitant metastatic sites of infection involving bones or joints should always raise a suspicion, concerning endovascular or endocardial infection. Neurologic expressions of disease such as stroke, focal neurologic deficits, transient psychological episodes, or cranial nerve dysfunction should also, when accompanied by fever or changing murmur or positive blood cultures, raise the possibility of infective endocarditis with cerebral involvement. Clearly, this should not be very surprising since fully a third of the patients who have classic infective endocarditis and no renal disease also have central nervous system expressions of their endocardial infection. An individual who has an extravascular site of infection and any one of these aforementioned signs should also be suspected of having endovascular involvement, and investigation via recurrent blood cultures, echocardiography, and close clinical scrutiny would be the minimum the clinician should apply in trying to assess the presence of infective endocarditis. In fact, because of the significance of this particular disease and the difficulty in making the diagnosis in this setting, it becomes apparent that the high mortality accompanying inadequately treated infective endocarditis must, of necessity, lead to overdiagnosis and overtreatment. The minimum features that should lead the physician to suspect the presence of endocarditis and possibly make its diagnosis should include: 1) the presence of a changing murmur unexplained by vascular overload; 2) fever; 3) positive blood culture, especially when associated with an access site infection; 4) metastatic infection; 5) embolic issue; 6) unexplained neurologic signs or symptoms; and 7) persistent extravascular sites of infection.

The problem becomes further compounded by recent debate concerning the significance of bacteremia originating and associated with a removable focus. Since *Staphylococcus aureus* is the organism most commonly involved in such transient bacteremic episodes and, indeed, is also the most common organism involved in infective endocarditis, such a debate takes on great significance for the physician managing the patient with chronic renal failure. Since the review by Wilson and Hamburger in 1957,[6] the association of *S. aureus* bacteremia and subsequent infective endocarditis has been well accepted. *S. aureus* bacteremia and resultant infective endocarditis have been associated with removable infected intravenous devices.[7] In a review of 21 patients with *S. aureus* bacteremia associated with infected intravenous devices, at least 8 of these individuals developed confirmed infective endocarditis and it was suspected that others might have also been afflicted. The review by Iannini and Crossly[8] emphasizing abbreviated therapy for *S. aureus* bacteremia when associated with a removable focus of infection suggests that infective endocarditis is a very uncommon phenomenon among individuals in whom a clearly definable and removable focus of infection can be found. Obviously peripheral intravenous catheters, central venous pressure devices, transvenous pacemakers, and dialysis shunts are examples of the types of devices encountered in this particular review. However, their numbers are small, especially when it comes to individuals on hemodialysis. If one finds an access site infection, it can be removed and only two weeks of therapy may be required in order to minimize the risk of infective endocarditis to the patient. The paper by Nolan and Beaty[9] on *S. aureus* bacteremia and its current clinical patterns also raises the intriguing question of the risk of developing subsequent infective endocarditis. They reviewed 140 episodes of bacteremia, 105 were given specific attention for the purpose of their paper, 63 of these individuals had a focus of infection that could be defined, and the remaining 42 failed to have a definable portal of entry or focus of infection. Noteworthy was the fact that if an identifiable focus of infection could be located, these individuals had a negligible risk of developing infective endocarditis. Whereas in the group with no primary focus of infection and associated staphylococcal bacteremia, the risk of infective endocarditis was exceedingly high. These authors did not present extensive experience with individuals on chronic hemodialysis and access site infections with *S. aureus* and ensuing bacteremia. Therefore, one cannot confidently conclude that in hemodialysis focal bacteremia there is a limited risk of developing subsequent infective endocarditis. Since Nolan and Beatty[9] also found a 21 percent morality associated with *S. aureus* bacteremia and serious disease, one has to approach the hemodialysis patient with associated staphylococcal bacteremia with great respect and a very strong suspicion that infective endocarditis might indeed result. Until better criteria can be devised to define deep and serious infection, treatment for infective endocarditis is probably indicated.

Because this is a major diagnostic and therapeutic problem and because therapy consisting of 4 to 6 weeks of parentally delivered antibiotic is the custom, other investigators have turned their attention to defining *serious* staphylococcal bacteremia. The work of Tuazon and

Sheagren[10] and others [11] discusses the presence of teichoic acid antibodies in response to staphylococcal infection. These authors have established that the presence of high titers of teichoic acid antibody in the serum of individuals with documented staphylococcal bacteremia suggests that deep seated significant infection exists. Clearly, this is not pathognomonic for infective endocarditis, but may also be found in osteomyelitis and other deep body sites of infection. Nonetheless, the higher the titer of these antibodies, the presence of specific immunoglobulin G antibody, the presence of an access site infection especially if other factors are present (see p. 177), lead to the conclusion that infective endocarditis is probably present and such individuals most assuredly should be committed to an ensuing course of therapy.

MANAGEMENT

The therapy of infective endocarditis, or any other bacterial infection for that matter, in the presence of chronic renal insufficiency differs somewhat from that in a patient with normal renal function. Since the majority of antimicrobials are handled at least in part by renal mechanisms, some modification of dosage and even some restrictions on drug selection become necessary.

In the individual on chronic hemodialysis with unknown septicemia or suspected infective endocarditis, initial therapy should be instituted according to the selections listed in Table 1. Our first choice of therapy would be nafcillin plus an amimoglycoside—either gentamicin or tobramycin or amikacin. One might substitute oxacillin and methicillin for the nafcillin in this regimen. The reasons for this selection include the overwhelming likelihood that S. aureus will be present and hence the semisynthetic penicillin which is resistant to staphylococcal peni-

TABLE 1. Initial therapy for infective
endocarditis in hemodialysis patients

I—Nafcillin (oxacillin, methicillin)
plus
Gentamicin (tobramycin, amikacin)
or
II—Vancomycin
plus
Gentamicin (tobramycin, amikacin)
or
III—Cephalothin (cefamandole, cefoxitin)
plus
Gentamicin (tobramycin, amikacin)

cillinase; also the likelihood that other gram-positive cocci, including enterococci, will be present against which nafcillin has a significant antimicrobial activity and in the presence of an aminoglycoside such as gentamicin (or tobramycin or amikacin) will have the significant likelihood of being synergistically active. The use of an aminoglycosidic antibiotic is also necessary at least initially to cover the possibility of a gram-negative bacillus causing the patient's infection. In institutions in which there is a significant incidence of gentamicin and/or tobramycin resistance among the gram-negative bacilli identified, then amikacin would be the aminoglycoside antibiotic of choice. Nafcillin and oxacillin which are capable of significant hepatic excretory pathways require no modification in the presence of chronic renal failure and so would be preferred to methicillin in such a combination regimen. In the event that the patient is allergic to penicillin, then vancomycin plus an aminoglycoside would be the therapy of choice. This regimen also will cover staphylococci including penicillinase producers and those resistant to nafcillin plus enterococci and, with the addition of an aminoglycocidic antibiotic, will also cover enteric gram-negative bacilli plus pseudomonads until the infectious organism can be thoroughly identified. A cephalosporinic acid derivative or a cefamycin derivative plus an aminoglycoside is listed in third place because there is a deficiency in its activity against the enterococci. For the most commonly encountered microorganisms in this clinical setting however, even in the presence of penicillin allergy, such a combination would most likely be effective.

Once the specific infectious organism is identified in any given patient, more appropriate and specific choices in antibiotic selection can be made. Table 2 lists some of the commonly encountered microorganisms and the antibiotics that would be preferred in diminishing order of preference to be employed against each one. As noted in Table 2, drugs useful against S. aureus include nafcillin, the cephalosporins, vancomycin, and clindamycin. In the case of penicillin allergy or in the presence of tolerance to semisynthetic penicillins, cephalosporinic acid derivatives of the first generation, including cephalothin, cephradine, and cephapirin, would appear to be logical alternatives. Because of persistence in the blood stream and the ability to give dosing on a less frequent basis, vancomycin might also be seriously considered as a second or even a first choice with S. aureus infective endocarditis in patients suffering from chronic renal insufficiency. Because of its ability to be excreted via the liver and the possibilities of being administered both parenterally and orally, clindamycin might also be considered in the therapy of S. aureus, although at present therapeutic outcome would suggest that this is not as good a choice as the aforementioned drugs.

TABLE 2. Antibiotic preferences for treatment of specific pathogens causing infective endocarditis in renal failure patients

Microbe	Antibiotics
Staphylococcus aureus	Nafcillin (oxacillin)
	Methicillin
	Cephalothin (cephapirin, cephradine)
	Vancomycin (clindamycin)
Staphylococcus epidermidis	Nafcillin (oxacillin)*
	Vancomycin
	Cephalothin, cephradine, cephapirin
Enterococcus	Penicillin G plus gentamicin
	or
	Ampicillin plus gentamicin
	or
	Vancomycin plus gentamicin
Other Streptococci	Penicillin G
	Vancomycin
	Cephalothin
	(Clindamycin)
Escherichia coli	Ampicillin
	Cephalothin[†] (cephradine or cephapirin)
	Cefamandole (or cefoxitin)
	Gentamicin (tobramycin or amikacin)
Klebsiella pneumoniae	Cefamandole or
	Cefoxitin[‡]
	Cephalothin
	plus
	Gentamicin (or tobramycin or amikacin)
Pseudomonas aeruginosa	Ticarcillin (or carbenicillin)
	plus
	Tobramycin (or gentamicin or amikacin)

In selected instances, the addition of polymyxin B or rifampin might be useful.
NOTE: Two new third generation cephalosporin antibiotics
      LY 127935 and HR 756 might prove more useful in this
      setting when available.

Diphtheroids	Vancomycin
	plus
	Aminoglycosides

*If resistant to methicillin then vancomycin plus an aminoglycoside or other combinations discussed in the text will be indicated.

†If resistant to cephalothin but susceptible to cefamandole or cefoxitin.

‡If susceptible to cephalothin then use cephalothin or cephradine or cephapirin.

The synergistic effect of an aminoglycosidic antibiotic in combination with another agent against *S. aureus* is still a matter of debate. Preliminary data suggest that although killing is more rapid, the resultant cure rate is no different. Further information and the results of studies currently underway will provide us with additional information concerning two drug therapy for *S. aureus* infective endocarditis.

Staphylococcus epidermidis poses a much more complex problem in chemotherapy. If susceptible to penicillin G or the semisynthetic penicillin derivatives with very low minimum bactericidal concentration (MBC), then these drugs alone will probably be sufficient. Increasingly however, we see a marked variation in the susceptibility of *S. epidermidis* for a variety of antibiotics. Methicillin resistance is not an uncommon occurrence and laboratory results might indicate methicillin resistance and cephalothin susceptibility. However, it would be advisable to disregard this information and not treat these individuals with a cephalosporin antibiotic. This is because the killing concentration (MBC) necessary for such strains is usually extremely high. Our first choice in this setting is vancomycin, very often in combination with either rifampin or erythromycin pending the outcome of more specific tube dilution sensitivity tests.

Against the enterococci, the combination of penicillin plus an aminoglycoside, such as gentamicin or ampicillin plus gentamicin or, in the case of penicillin allergy, vancomycin plus gentamicin or another aminoglycoside, is the appropriate approach. When streptococci other than enterococci are present, penicillin G alone or vancomycin alone or a cephalosporinic acid alone would be the appropriate first choice antimicrobials to employ.

Therapy for gram-negative bacilli is also a complex issue. Among susceptible *Escherichia coli*, ampicillin would be the drug of choice. If ampicillin resistance and cephalothin susceptibilty exists, then cephalothin or cephradine or cephapirin would be acceptable therapeutic choices. Nonetheless, the increasing incidence of resistance among coliform bacteria to first generation cephalosporins will mandate therapy with cefamandole or cefoxitin. In the presence of gram-negative enteric rod endocarditis, many researchers would also suggest concomitant therapy with an aminoglycoside such as gentamicin, tobramycin, or amikacin because of potential synergy. However, no data are currently available on the value of two-drug therapy for infective endocarditis due to coliforms and it appears that no advantage acrues using a single beta lactam antibiotic with a low MBC for the organism.

With Klebsiella, the initial therapeutic choice would be cefamandole or cefoxitin, especially since we are increasingly encountering cephalothin resistance within this genus. If, however, we find that the organism in question is susceptible with a low MBC to cephalothin, then this certainly would be a suitable therapeutic alternative. The need for a second drug, in particular an aminoglycoside, is even more controversial here, but the use of a second antibiotic with the more tenacious Klebsiella genus is appropriate. In addition to the cephalosporinic acid derivative, gentamicin, tobramycin or amikacin can be added.

Pseudomonas aeruginosa also poses grave therapeutic problems in any setting in which it is encountered. Optimal therapy would appear to be ticarcillin (or carbenicillin) plus tobramycin (or gentamicin or amikacin). In the presence of chronic renal insufficiency, the increased propensity toward thrombocytopathy and coagulopathy with increasing large dose ticarcillin or carbenicillin therapy is a potential handicap. Should these difficulties ensue, one must of necessity lower the dose of the penicillin derivative and rely predominantly on the aminoglycosidic antibiotic for inhibition of the organism causing infection. In some settings, because of lack of synergy or inability to sterilize the blood stream and the absence of a removable infectious focus, the addition of a third agent such as polymyxin B or rifampin might become necessary. Noteworthy on the horizon are two third generation cephalosporinic acid derivatives notably LY 127935 and HR756 which have very broad spectrums of cidal activity, including Pseudomonas aeruginosa, which might prove to be much more useful than currently available drugs.

The monitoring of therapy for infective endocarditis is particularly significant in renal impairment. The determination of the minimum concentration of antibiotic necessary to both inhibit and kill the infective microorganism is essential.[12] This is particularly true of the patient with renal insufficiency in whom it will be necessary, in many instances, to limit the amount of antimicrobial agent delivered to the patient. The principal therefore is to determine the MIC/MBC of the infecting microorganisms to the antibiotic agent selected and potential alternative therapeutic choices. Subsequent determinations of serum antibacterial activity by measuring serum bactericidal levels should be carried out on a weekly basis with the therapeutic end-point being a serum MBC of ≥ 1 to 16 dilutions.

Another problem encountered is the need for determining the actual blood levels of antimicrobial agents that accompany a given dosage schedule in these patients. This may be unnecessary or only of academic importance among such agents as the penicillin derivatives in which a wide therapeutic toxicity margin is present, but becomes more critical among potentially toxic drugs. Even in the presence of renal failure, the aminoglycosidic antibiotics have extra renal toxicity. Vancomycin is another agent whose therapeutic blood level should not be significantly exceeded because of the potential for eighth nerve toxicity. Once a therapeutic concentration of antimicrobial agent is present in the blood stream, further dosage modifications must consider the kinetics of that agent in the particular patient involved. The alternatives for maintaining adequate therapeutic blood levels are either increasing the frequency of dosing and diminishing the amount given at each interval or increasing the dose given and lengthening the interval between doses. At present, it is not clear whether one of these options is superior.

References 13 through 32 discuss the clinical pharmacokinetics of various drugs in renal insufficiency with particular emphasis on antimicrobial agents. The reader is referred to these particular references and to Table 3 for details regarding dosage modification and usage in patients with varying degrees of renal dysfunction. Some brief comments about specific groups of antimicrobials will follow.

The Penicillins

As a group, the penicillin antibiotics are eliminated primarily via glomerular filtration with tubular secretion. In the presence of renal insufficiency, hepatic metabolism and biliary tract excretion may account for a significant portion of the penicillin derivate removed from the body. In spite of a large therapeutic toxicity margin, the large concentrations of penicillins required for the therapy of infective endocarditis may lead to toxicity. Bryan and Stone [16] have derived a nomogram that provides a simple method for achieving a desired level of penicillin G concentration in patients with renal insufficiency as follows: the maintenance of penicillin G in units per 24 hours is defined by the product of penicillin clearance in ml/min x the desired penicillin concentration in μg/ml x 2300. Hemodialysis clears penicillin G at approximately 40 ml/min so that 500,000 units should be given for every 6 hours of dialysis to replace expected loses. Because of the large quantities of sodium and potassium contained in penicillin derivatives, potassium or sodium imbalance may be exaggerated in the patient with renal insufficiency. The approximate sodium and potassium concentrations of several penicillin derivatives are included in Table 4.

A noteworthy exception to the glomerular filtration and tubular secretion method of excretion for penicillin derivatives is the excretion of nafcillin and isoxazolyl penicillins. These include nafcillin, cloxacillin, dicloxacillin and oxacillin. These have such significant hepatobiliary excretion that dosing is essentially unmodified in the anephric state and in patients on dialysis. Since in general the metabolic pathway via the liver and hepatobiliary tree for other penicillins is less than that for penicillin G, more significant dosage reduction is necessary for these other derivatives. For example, 17 percent of penicillin G is metabolized via

TABLE 3. Indicated modifications in antimicrobial therapy in renal failure.

Drug	Degree of Renal Failure		Hemodialysis (additional change due to dialysis)
	Mild	Severe	
Penicillin G	NC	2 mu q6h	Add $^1/_4$ dose postdialysis
Nafcillin	NC	NC	NC
Methicillin	NC	30% reduction	15–20% reduction
Cloxacillin	NC	NC	NC
Dicloxacillin	NC	NC	NC
Oxacillin	NC	NC	NC
Carbenicillin	2–3 gm q4h	1 gm q6h	Add 1–2 gm
Ticarcillin	2 gm q4h	1 gm q6h	Add 1–2 gm postdialysis
Ampicillin	NC	30% reduction	Add $^1/_4$ dose postdialysis
Amoxicillin	NC	50–60% reduction	Add $^1/_4$ dose postdialysis
Cephalothin	NC	1 gm q12h	Add 1 gm postdialysis
Cephapirin	NC	1 gm q12h	Add 1 gm postdialysis
Cephradine	$^1/_2$ dose reduction	500 mg/24 hr	Add 500 mg postdialysis
Cephaloridine	Avoid	Avoid	Avoid
Cephalexin	$^1/_2$ dose reduction	500 mg/24 hr	Add 500 mg postdialysis
Cefoxitin	NC	1 gm/12 hr	Add 1 gm postdialysis
Cefamandole	NC	1 gm/12 hr	Add 1 gm postdialysis
Cefazolin	$^1/_2$ gm/12 hr	500 mg/24 hr	Add $^1/_2$ gm postdialysis
Gentamicin	$1-1.75$ mg/kg/ Creat = dose q8h	$\dfrac{1-1.75\,mg/kg}{Creat}$ q8h	Load then 1 mg/kg postdialysis
Tobramycin	"	"	"
Amikacin	$\dfrac{7.5\,mg/kg}{Creat}$ q12h	"	Load then 7.5 mg/kg postdialysis
Clindamycin	NC	300 mg q8h	NC
Vancomycin	1 gm/day	1 gm/week	1 gm/week
Chloramphenicol	NC	NC	NC
Rifampin	NC	300 mg/day	300 mg/day
Amphotericin B	0.5 mg/kg/24 hr		same
5-fluorcytosine	25–50 mg/kg' 12 hr	25–50 mg/kg' 24 hr	25–50 mg/kg postdialysis

TABLE 4. Sodium/potassium content of some penicillin derivatives

Drug	Sodium	Potassium
Penicillin G (per million units)	1.7 mEq	1.4 mEq
Ampicillin (per gram)	3.4 mEq	
Oxacillin (per gram)	3.1 mEq	
Methicillin	55 μg/gm	
Carbenicillin	4.7 mEq/gm	
Ticarcillin	4.7 mEq/gm	

the liver; 12 percent of ampicillin; 5 percent of carbenicillin. Dialysis does not remove significant quantities of the isoxazolyl penicillins or methicillin. Up to 30 percent of the body stores of other penicillin derivatives may be removed after dialysis and therefore these must be replaced after each hemodialysis in order to maintain therapeutic levels. Peritoneal dialysis results in no more than 15 percent removal when maximal efficiency of this pathway is present for the extraction of penicillin from the body.

Cephalosporinic Acid Derivatives

All of the cephalosporinic acid derivatives are excreted via renal mechanisms, i.e., glomerular filtration and/or tubular secretion. As a result, dosage modification is necessary for any creatinine clearance of less than 20 ml/min. In the case of cephalothin, cephradine, cephapirin, cefamandole, and cefoxitin, a loading dose of between 1 and 2 gm followed by a maintenance dose of ¼ to ½ the loading dose every 8 to 12 hours should provide satisfactory therapeutic levels in most circumstances. Six to eight hours of hemodialysis should remove 30 to 50 percent of the body stores of the cephalosporins whereas peritoneal dialysis will remove only 10 to 30 percent of the body stores after 24 to 36 hours of therapy. These must be replaced following dialysis. It is our practice with cefamandole and cefoxitin that, following the loading dose, 1 gm every 12 hours be administered to the patient while undergoing hemodialytic therapy with followup measurement of the serum bactericidal activity to insure that, in fact, we have achieved an adequate therapeutic level.

Aminoglycosides

Aminoglycosidic antibiotics are excreted almost entirely via renal mechanism. Significant dosage reduction is mandated for all of these drugs. This must be further modified by serial measurements of serum antibiotic levels in order to guarantee that in any given individual a therapeutic level is maintained. Adjustments for dosing aminoglycosides in the presence of renal dysfunction can be accomplished by many mechanisms. It is our recommendation that the loading dose for the particular individual be divided by the creatinine and delivered at the usual interval of 8 to 12 hours depending on which aminoglycoside is selected (see Table 3).

Hemodialysis removes 30 to 50 percent of the body stores of the aminoglycoside drugs, whereas 24 hours of peritoneal dialysis will remove only 10 to 25 percent of the drug. Accordingly, it is recommended that supplemental doses be provided following each period of dialysis.

Miscellaneous Agents

This category includes clindamycin, with can be given in full therapeutic doses in mild renal failure, but in severe renal insufficiency should be reduced to 300 to 600 mg every 8 hr. There would be no further reduction in the presence of hemodialysis. Vancomycin may be administered in mild renal dysfunction in maximal doses of 1gm/day, and in severe renal dysfunction or anuria 1 gm/week is probably sufficient. This dose is not altered by hemodialysis. Chloramphenicol which has inconsequential renal excretion and is predominantly excreted via hepatobiliary pathways would require no dosage modification in the presence of renal insufficiency. Attention has to be given to the marrow depressant effects of this drug and the fact that metabolites of chloramphenicol will accumulate more rapidly in the presence of renal failure. Although these metabolites are less effective as antibacterial products, they do contribute to the marrow toxicity of this particular agent.

Rifampin

Rifampin as an adjunctive drug in the therapy of both gram-positive coccal as well as selected gram-negative bacillary endocarditis would require no modification in mild renal dysfuntion. In the presence of severe renal dysfunction, maximal doses of 300 mg per day are suggested. In view of the inadequacy of available information, 300 mg daily should be continued in the presence of hemodialysis, although we feel that we may be continually underdosing such patients. In the presence of rifampin employed as an adjunctive agent, it becomes necessary to measure serum antibacterial activity to assess whether or not the synergy demonstrated in in vitro studies has occurred in vivo.

Duration of Therapy

The duration of therapy for infective endocarditis is still uncertain even currently. Guidelines have been published by many authors based upon the predisposing factors with a cardiovascular prosthesis and the particular microorganism involved. In general, therapeutic duration is from 4 to 6 weeks and most authorities agree that it should be delivered parenterally throughout the course of therapy. The patient in chronic renal failure undergoing maintenance hemodialysis provides a unique opportunity for the retention of certain antimicrobial agents, i.e., vancomycin and aminoglycosidic drugs. Appropriate therapy for the infecting agent might permit the individual, when clinically stable and improved, to leave the hospital and have the drug administered at varying intervals during their routine hemodialysis sessions. This obviously is something that can be done only at the discretion of the individual clinician, and serum antibacterial activity must be monitored throughout the course of treatment to be certain that sufficient levels of antibacterial activity are maintained. Serial blood cultures should be performed during the course of therapy despite the defervesence of the patient and apparent clinical improvement. This is particularly so among patients with chronic renal insufficiency in whom modification of the host response might be due to renal failure and not to therapeutic benefit.

REFERENCES

1.   Nsouli, K.A., Lazarus, M., Schoenbaum, S.C. et al.: Bacteremic infection in hemodialysis. Arch. Intern. Med. 139:1255, 1979.
2.   Cross, A.S., and Steigbigel, R.T.: Infective endocarditis and access site infections in patients on hemodialysis. Medicine 55:453, 1976.
3.   Leonard, A., Raij, L., and Shapiro, F.L.: Bacterial endocarditis in regularly dialyzed patients. Kidney Inter. 4:407, 1973.
4.   Leonard, A., Raij, L., et al.: Experience with endocarditis in a large kidney disease program. Trans. Am. Soc. Artif. Int. Organs 19:298, 1973.
5.   King, L.H., et al.: Bacterial endocarditis in chronic hemodialysis patients; a complication more common than previously suspected. Surgery 69:554, 1971.
6.   Wilson, R., and Hamburger, M.: Fifteen years experience with staphylococcus septicemia in a large city hospital—analysis of fifty-five cases in the Cincinnati General Hospital 1940–1954. Am. J. Med. 22:437, 1957.
7.   Watanakunakorn, C., and Baird, M.: S. aureus bactermia and endocarditis associated with a removable focus of infection. Am. J. Med. 63:253, 1977.
8.   Iannini, P.B., and Crossley, K.: Therapy of Staphylococcus aureus bacteremia associated with a removable focus of infection. Ann. Intern. Med. 84:558, 1976.
9.   Nolan, C.M., and Beaty, H.N.: Staphylococcus aureus bacteremia: current clinical patterns. Am. J. Med. 60:495, 1976.

10. Tuazon, C.U., and Sheagren, J.N.: Teichoic acid antibodies in the diagnosis of serious infections with *Staphylococcus aureus*. Ann. Intern. Med. 84:543, 1976.

11. Wheat, L.J., Kohler, R.B., and White, A.: Solid-phase radioimmunoassay for immunoglobulin G *Staphylococcus aureus* antibody in serious staphylococcal infection. Ann. Intern. Med. 89:467, 1978.

12. Schwartz, A.R.: What is adequate therapy for infective endocarditis? *in* Lowenthal, D.T., and Major, D.A. (ed.): Clinical Therapeutics. Grune and Stratton, New York, 1978, p. 315.

13. Welling, P.G., and Craig, W.A.: Pharmacokinetics in disease states modifying renal function, *in* Benet, L.Z. (ed.): The Effect of Disease States on Drug Pharmacokinetics. Amer. Pharmacology Assoc., Washington, D.C., 1976, p. 155.

14. Fabre, J., and Balant, L.: Renal failure, drug pharmacokinetics and drug action. Clinical Pharmacokinetics 1:99, 1976.

15. Bennett, W.M. et al.: Guidelines for drug therapy in renal failure. Ann. Intern. Med. 86:754, 1977.

16. Bryan, C.S., and Stone, W.J.: "Comparably massive" penicillin G therapy in renal failure. Ann. Intern. Med. 82:189, 1975.

17. Appel, G.B., and Neu, H.C.: The nephrotoxicity of antimicrobial agents. N. Engl. J. Med. 296:663, 1977.

18. Marcy, S.M., and Klein, J.O.: The isoxazoyl penicillins: oxacillin, cloxacillin and dicloxacillin. Med. Clin. North Am. 54:1127, 1970.

19. Hoffman, T.A., Cestero, R., and Bullock, W.E.: Pharmacodynamics of carbenicillin in hepatic and renal failure. Ann. Intern. Med. 73:173, 1970.

20. Gombos, E.A., Katz, S., Fedorko, J., et al.: Dialysis properties of newer antimicrobial agents. Antimicrob. Agents Chemother. 4:373, 1964.

21. Ruedy, J.: The effects of peritoneal dialysis on the physiological disposition of oxacillin, ampicillin and tetracycline in patients with renal disease. Canad. Med. Assoc. J. 94:257, 1966.

22. Kirby, W.M., DeMaine, J.B., and Serrill, W.S.: Pharmacokinetics of the cephalosporins in healthy volunteers and uremic patients. Postgrad. Med. J. 47:Suppl.:41, 1971.

23. Venuto, R.C. and Plaut, M.E.: Cephalothin handling in patients undergoing hemodialysis. Antimicrob. Agents Chemother. 10:50, 1970.

24. Buck, A.C., and Cohen, S.L.: Absorption of antibiotics during peritoneal dialysis in patients with renal failure. J. Clin. Pathol. 21:88, 1968.

25. Culter, R.E., Gyselynck, A.M., Fleet, W.P., et al.: Correlation of serum creatinine concentrations and gentamicin half-life. JAMA 219:1037, 1972.

26. Lockwood, W.R. and Bower, J.D.: Tobramycin and gentamicin concentrations in the serum of normal and anephric patients. Antimicrob. Agents Chemother. 3:125, 1973.

27. Cimino, J.E., and Tierno, P.M., Jr.: Hemodialysis properties of clindamycin (7-chloro 7-deoxylincomycin). Appl. Microbiol. 17:446, 1969.

28. Lindholm, D.D., and Murray, J.S.: Persistance of vancomycin in blood during renal failure and its treatment by hemodialysis. N. Engl. J. Med. 274:1074, 1966.

29. Jenne, J.W., and Beggs, W.H.: Correlation of *in vitro* and *in vivo* kinetics with clinical use of isoniazid, ethambutol and rifampin. Ann. Rev. Resp. Dis. 107:1013, 1973.

30. Bindschadler, D.D., and Bennett, J.E.: A pharmacologic guide to the clinical use of amphotericin B. J. Infect. Dis. 120:427, 1969.

31.   Block, E.R., Bennett, J.E., Livoti, L.G., et al.: Flucytosine and amphotericin B: hemodialysis effects on the plasma concentrations and clearance studies in man. Ann. Intern. Med. 80:613, 1974.
32.   Bryan, C.S. and Stone, W.J.: Antimicrobial dosage in renal failure: a unifying nomogram. Clin. Neph. 7:81, 1977.

11

CARDIAC SURGERY IN CHRONIC RENAL FAILURE

Inder P. Goel, M.D. and Eldred D. Mundth, M.D.

The need for cardiac surgical procedures in patients with chronic renal failure is infrequent, but the incidence has increased significantly over the last 5 years. Since the initiation of hemodialysis 17 years ago for management of chronic renal failure, the number of patients enrolled in hospital and home programs has steadily increased to its present level of approximately 30,000 patients annually. This number is expected to double over the next two decades. Two important clinical facts have become apparent with this experience: 1) There has been a steady improvement in prolongation of life in this group of patients with the expected yearly survival rate now being in the 90 percent range. 2) This group of patients can develop cardiac disease unassociated with chronic renal failure or develop cardiac disorders related to chronic renal failure and uremia or as a complication of hemodialysis which may require surgical treatment. The most frequently seen cardiovascular disorders requiring surgical intervention are: 1) uremic pericarditis; 2) subacute bacterial endocarditis; 3) accelerated coronary artery disease.

UREMIC PERICARDITIS

Pericarditis associated with chronic renal failure and uremia was first recognized and reported by Richard Bright in 1836.[3] The clinical features have been described in Chapters 4, 5, and 6. Hemodynamically significant pericardial effusion and tamponade have been recognized with increasing frequency. In many instances, uremic effusions will respond to an increased frequency of hemodialysis, but on occasion the effusion will continue and progress and produce significant hemodynamic impairment requiring emergency surgical intervention. Surgical interventions that may be required include: 1) pericardiocentesis; 2) percardial window; and 3) pericardiectomy.

A recent review of the results of management of uremic pericarditis from a large volume hemodialysis program indicated that conservative management with more frequent dialysis and repeated pericardiocentesis was sufficient in nearly all patients.[8]

The authors found an incidence of 6.9 percent of clinically significant pericardial effusion. All of these patients were managed initially by increasing the frequency of dialysis and 63 percent responded to this mode of treatment. In 37 percent pericardiocentesis was required for relief of pericardial effusion. Only 5.5 percent of patients who developed pericardial effusion failed to respond to this form of management and required more definitive operative procedures including one partial pericardiectomy and two subtotal pericardiectomies later in the clinical course. Particularly in patients with severe physiologic abnormalities associated with uremia, this more conservative approach seems warranted as an initial mode of management of uremic pericardial effusion. The potential complications of pericardiocentesis include pneumothorax, pneumoperitoneum, costochondritis, and myocardial puncture, but these are rare.

Some groups, however, have advised a limited pericardial window using a subxyphoid approach or through an anterolateral pleuro-pericardial approach for all patients who do not respond to increased frequency of hemodialysis. Clinical experience has shown that whatever surgical means are used to deal with life threatening cardiac tamponade due to pericardial effusion, the late results are very gratifying.

SUBACUTE BACTERIAL ENDOCARDITIS

Bacterial endocarditis is not a rare complication in a regular dialysis program. The age and sex distribution reflects that of the program itself and the complication occurs more commonly one to two years after the initiation of dialysis; it usually occurs as a complication secondary to access infection. The incidence of subacute bacterial endocarditis in one large dialysis unit series was reported as 2.7 percent.[10]

Various factors have been identified as being the predisposing causes of subacute bacterial endocarditis in the dialysis group of patients: 1) increased cardiovascular stress associated with an arteriovenous fistula; 2) environmental changes or endocrine alterations which may predispose the valvular endothelium to bacterial infection; 3) persistence or recurrence of bacteremia when an arteriovenous fistula exists; 4) change in immunologic and other natural defenses to fight infection.

Any valve may be involved, but the most common is the aortic valve followed by the mitral and rarely the tricuspid valve.

A variety of infecting organisms has been cultured from these patients, including *Staphylococcus aureus, Staphylococcus epidermidis, Streptococcus viridans,* enterococcus, Corynebacterium, and *Pseudomonas aeruginosa.* The most common infecting organisms are *Staph. aureus, Staph. epidermidis,* and *strep. viridans.*

Once the patients develop subacute bacterial endocarditis and the specific infecting organisms are isolated, they are treated with an appropriate intensive parenteral antibiotic regimen. However, some patients may develop significant hemodynamic complications or become resistant to antibiotic treatment and require surgical intervention by way of surgical replacement of the affected valve. The results of surgery for bacterial endocarditis in uremic patients can be expected to be reasonably acceptable. Overall management is complicated by the presence of renal insufficiency, but satisfactory results have been achieved by units experienced in the management of this type of patient.

ACCELERATED CORONARY ARTERY DISEASE

It has been shown that the incidence of atherosclerotic coronary artery disease may be higher in patients with chronic renal failure as compared to normal and hypertensive groups of patients of comparable age and rates similar to those found in Type II hyperlipoproteinemia.[11] (See Chapters 1 and 6 for discussion.)

After the first few years of dialysis the cumulative probability of dying from all causes parallels the increasing probability of dying from an atherosclerotic complication.[11] The six year incidence of coronary artery disease for patients on hemodialysis is about 2.5 times that for an older group of men with hypercholesterolemia reported in the Framingham study.[11]

Coronary artery bypass surgery is an acceptable form of treatment for both stable and unstable angina pectoris in patients without kidney disease. There are, however, few published reports of coronary artery bypass surgery in patients with associated terminal renal failure.

Thus far, 27 patients undergoing chronic dialysis or post-transplantation have been reported in the literature to have safely undergone myocardial revascularization, some of them also having valve replacement at the same time.[13-27] Our experience and collective experience from literature indicates that these patients can undergo angiography and coronary artery bypass surgery at an increased but acceptable risk. The operation benefits patients with end-stage renal failure and severe ischemic heart disease by relieving angina and improving their level of activity. It is unclear whether survival is improved for these patients.

CARDIAC SURGERY IN CHRONIC RENAL FAILURE

Performing open heart surgery in patients with chronic renal failure can be challenging. Grossly abnormal physiology due to chronic renal failure may create problems during and after operation which are difficult to manage, therefore, a thorough preoperative evaluation is essential.

Coagulation and platelet function are abnormal in end-stage renal disease.[28-30] The association of bleeding tendency with uremia has been recognized for at least a century.[28] Platelet counts are generally normal but may be decreased 16 to 53 percent below normal in some cases. The most common abnormality is related to abnormal platelet function despite normal platelet morphology and quantity. The functional consequences are: prolonged bleeding time, decreased platelet retention on glass beads, decreased collagen or ADP-induced aggregation, and decreased function of platelet Factor III activity.

Although sufficient followup data are not available, in spite of the coagulopathy, one could expect that progression of atherosclerosis in bypass coronary arteries and in the bypass conduits may be at an increased rate in uremic patients. Followup angiographic study will be necessary to ascertain the prognosis of chronic renal failure patients undergoing coronary bypass surgery. Short term results have been encouraging with the great majority of patients experiencing excellent functional benefit.

In patients with chronic renal failure, careful preoperative preparation is necessary before cardiac surgery is performed. In most cases, dialysis should be instituted the day before surgery so as to keep the fluid and electrolyte balance and BUN levels as near normal as possible. This will, in many cases, forestall the necessity of early postoperative dialysis when the chest tubes are still in place. If the hematocrit is less than 20 percent, it is desirable to raise the hematocrit value to 30 percent, particularly in patients undergoing open heart surgery. This will enable the patients to better withstand blood loss if hemodilution is used in priming for cardiopulmonary bypass. A slow transfusion of packed cells can be used for this purpose: great caution must be exercised in patients with cardiac decompensation and oliguria. Fresh blood should be ordered whenever possible for intraoperative and postoperative use to avoid higher potassium content of bank blood over 5 days old; also fresh platelet concentrate should be ordered for postoperative use.

Intraoperatively, fresh blood should be used for priming the pump if the patient's hematocrit is below 30 percent. No exogenous potassium should be used and frequent determinations of potassium should be done. Fluid administration must be carefully monitored. Minimal amounts of noncolloid fluid can be administered, and consequently the fluid vehicle for administration of drugs during the course of surgery must be minimized. No more than a total of 100 ml/hour noncolloid fluid should be administered. Appropriate blood volume adjustment can be instituted intraoperatively by simultaneous monitoring of the pulmonary capillary wedge pressure (utilizing the Swan-Ganz flow directed balloon tipped pulmonary artery catheter with a thermal sensor) or direct mean left atrial pressure, the central venous pressure, and hematocrit. It is most helpful in the management of patients with cardiac disease to also monitor the cardiac output serially using the relatively simple thermal dilution technique.* It is essential to maintain an adequate cardiac output intraoperatively without volume overload and in most instances this can be achieved readily using the approach described. Postoperatively, fresh blood and fresh platelets may be required for excessive bleeding.

A most important aspect of postoperative management is fluid and electrolyte balance. The most sensitive parameter of fluid balance, namely urine volume, may be nil. Thus, the postoperative use of left atrial pressure (left atrial pressure line inserted at the time of surgery) or Swan-Ganz pulmonary capillary wedge pressure, central venous pressure, pulse rate, blood pressure, tissue perfusion, and twice daily weights by use of metabolic weighing scales greatly assist in maintenance of proper fluid balance.

Electrolytes, in particular potassium, should be checked frequently in the immediate postoperative period. Parenteral fluids given during the early postoperative period should include fresh blood to match mediastinal drainage and to replace insensible losses with a crystalloid (10% dextrose in water) containing 500 to 700 ml in 24 hours. If there are other fluid losses, they should be replaced accordingly. Saline is generally not used unless there are gastrointestinal losses; as a rule potassium is not given. Vasopressors are given in concentrated solutions if necessary. Digitalis is given in half the maintenance dose. Despite rigid fluid restrictions, these patients may develop fluid overload particularly due to mobilization of fluid retained in the tissues (used for priming the pump) while on cardiopulmonary bypass. This may result in delayed pulmonary edema from mobilization of excess tissue fluid and necessitate prolonged respiratory support and repeated dialysis.

Besides fluid overload, the main indication for early postoperative dialysis is a rising potassium level, which can result in serious cardiac arrhythmias, particularly AV conduction delay or sinus arrest. Prophylactic use of ion exchange resin (Kayexalate) enemas twice a day starting on the first postoperative day sometimes is helpful in preventing a rapid rise in potassium level. Generally speaking, dialysis is needed by the third or fourth postoperative day; early dialysis may be needed if the serum potassium rises to 6 mEq/liter. Peritoneal dialysis is preferable to hemodialysis during the first postoperative week. This avoids the abrupt hemodynamic changes and bleeding or clotting problems which may be encountered with hemodialysis. Implantation of a peritoneal dialysis catheter, if not already present, at the end of the cardiac surgical procedure can save time and inconvenience later and is immediately available for dialysis should the need arise. One can switch to hemodialysis later in the postoperative course using "regional" heparinization initially and then full heparinization. Peritoneal dialysis may be contraindicated when accidental continuity of the thorax and/or pericardium has been created at operation or previous abdominal surgery has resulted in peritoneal adhesions. Additionally, where respiratory problems create serious difficulties postoperatively, one is limited in terms of the peritoneal exchange volume that can be used. In such circumstances, peritoneal dialysis may be of limited value and it may be necessary to use hemodialysis earlier.

ANTICOAGULATION

Whether chronic renal failure patients with prosthetic cardiac valves should be on long term anticoagulation is debatable. Because of abnormalities in the clotting mechanism, it may be argued that not only is anticoagulation unnecessary but also that it may increase the changes of spontaneous bleeding. On the other hand, uremic patients are known to develop acute thrombotic episodes, especially soon after termination of hemodialysis. There is no reason to believe that such a thrombotic process would spare involvement of prosthetic heart valves. Because of these considerations it is generally accepted that patients with prosthetic heart valves be placed on long term anticoagulants in the belief that it may be easier to control bleeding episodes with careful regulation of the warfarin dose and prothrombin time than to regulate problems related to thrombosis at the valve site and possible thromboembolic phenomena.

LONG-TERM PROPHYLACTIC ANTIBIOTIC COVERAGE

Because of the need for chronic hemodialysis, septicemia and bacterial endocarditis are constant threats (see Chap. 10). The presence of a foreign body such as a prosthetic cardiac valve causes additional concern. Use of prophylactic antibiotics for two months postoperatively has been recommended. However, long term use of prophylactic antibiotic therapy poses the danger of superinfection with resistant organisms.

Therefore, use of appropriate antibiotics is only recommended if there is an identified focus of infection.

CONCLUSION

Considering all the potential complications of open heart surgery in general and particularly in patients with chronic renal failure, the specific problems of bacterial endocarditis and long term anticoagulation make it debatable whether open heart surgery should be considered in these patients. The answer often is difficult. However, where cardiac surgery would normally be indicated, it frequently has been life saving in uremic patients and the short term results have been very encouraging.

REFERENCES

1. Cross, A.S., and Steigbigel, R.T.: Infective endocarditis and access site infections in patients on haemodialysis. Medicine 55:453, 1976.
2. Statistical reviews: dialysis, transplantation nephrology, in Morehead, J., Mion, E. and Baillod, R. (eds.): Proceedings of the European Dialysis and Transplantation Association, Vol. 12. Pittman, London, 1973, p. 11.
3. Bright, R.: Tabular view of the morbid appearances in 100 cases connected with albuminous urine with observations. Guy's Hosp. Rep. 1:380, 1836.
4. Baraet, A.L.: Pericarditis in chronic nephritis. Am. J. Med. Sci. 163:44, 1922.
5. Beandry, E., Nakamoto, S., and Koff, W.J.: Uraemic pericarditis and cardiac tamponade in chronic renal failure. Ann. Intern. Med. 64:990, 1966.
6. Richter, A.B., and O'Hare, J.P.: Heart in chronic glomerulonephritis. N. Engl. J. Med. 214:824, 1936.
7. Guild, W.R., Bray, G., and Merrill, J.P.: Hemopericardium with cardiac tamponade in chronic uraemia. N. Engl. J. Med. 257:230, 1957.
8. Kwasnik, E.M., Koster, K., Lazarus, J.M., et al.: Conservative management of uremic pericarditis effusions. J. Thorac. Cardiovasc. Surg. 76(5):629, 1978.
9. Schlein, E.M., Bartley, T.D., Spooner, G.R., et al.: A simple surgical approach to therapy of uremic pericarditis with tamponade. Ann. Thorac. Surg. 10(6):548, 1970.
10. Leonard, A., Raiz, L., and Shapiro, F.L.: Bacterial endocarditis in regularly dialyzed patients. Kidney Internat. 4:407, 1973.
11. Linder, A., Charra, B., Sherra, J.D., et al.: Accelerated atherosclerosis in prolonged maintenance hemodialysis. N. Engl. J. Med. 290(13):697, 1974.
12. Kannel, W.B., Dawber, T.R., Kagan, A., et al.: Factors of risk in the development of coronary artery disease: Six-year follow-up study: The Framingham Study. Ann. Intern. Med. 55:33, 1961.
13. Lansing, A.M., Masri, Z.H., Karalukulasingam, R., et al.: Angina during hemodialysis: treatment of coronary bypass graft. JAMA 232:736, 1975.
14. Crawford, F.A., Jr., Selby, J.H., Jr., Bower, J.D., et al.: Coronary revascularization in patients maintained on chronic hemodialysis. Circulation 56:684, 1977.
15. Sakurai, H., Ackad, A., Friedman, H.S., et al.: Aorto-coronary bypass graft surgery in a patient on home hemodialysis. Clin. Nephrol. 2:208, 1974.

16. Siegel, M.S., Norfleet, E.A., and Gitelman, H.J.: Coronary artery bypass surgery in a patient receiving hemodialysis. Arch. Intern. Med. 137:83, 1977.

17. Byrd, L.J., and Sullivan, J.F.: Successful coronary artery bypass in hemodialysis patients. J. Dialysis 2:33, 1978.

18. Beauchamp, G.D., Sharma, J.N., Crouch, T., et al.: Coronary bypass surgery after renal transplantation. Am. J. Cardiol. 37:1107, 1976.

19. Menzoian, J.O., Davis, R.C., Idelson, B.A., et al.: Coronary artery bypass surgery and renal transplantation: A case report. Ann. Surg. 179:63, 1974.

20. Kuehnel, E., Lundh, H., Bennett, W., et al.: Aortocoronary bypass surgery in patients with end-stage renal disease. Trans. Am. Soc. Artif. Intern. Organs 22:14, 1976.

21. Nakhjavan, F.K., Kahn, D., Rosenbaum, J., et al.: Aortocoronary vein graft surgery in a cadaver kidney transplant recipient. Arch. Intern. Med. 135: 1511, 1975.

22. Lansing, A.M., Leb, D.E., and Berman, L.B.: Cardiovascular surgery in end-stage renal failure. JAMA 204:682, 1968.

23. Rigot, S., Gilbert, L., Rothfield, E.L., et al.: Bacterial endocarditis with pulmonary edema necessitating mitral valve replacement in a hemodialysis-dependent patient. J. Thorac. Cardiovasc. Surg. 62:59, 1971.

24. Manhas, D.R., and Meredino, K.A.: The management of cardiac surgery in patients with chronic renal failure. J. Thorac. Cardiovasc. Surg. 63:235, 1972.

25. Haimov, M., Glabman, S., Schupak, E., et al.: General surgery in patients on maintenance hemodialysis. Ann. Surg. 179:863, 1974.

26. Posner, M.A., Reves, J.G., and Lell, W.A.: Aortic valve replacement in a hemodialysis-dependent patient: anesthetic considerations. Anesth. Analg. (Cleve.) 54:24, 1975.

27. Francis, G.S., Sharma, B., and Collins, A.J.: Coronary artery surgery in patients with end-stage renal disease. Ann. Intern. Med. 93:499, 1980.

28. Riesman, D.: Hemorrhages in the course of Bright's disease with special reference to the occurrence of a hemorrhagic diathesis of nephritic origin. Am. J. Med. Sci. 134:709, 1907.

29. Rath, C.E., Mailliand, J.A., and Schreiner, G.E.: Bleeding tendency in uremia. N. Engl. J. Med. 257(17):808, 1958.

30. Horowitz, H.I., Cohen, B.D., Martinez, P., et al.: Defective ADP-induced platelet factor 3 activation in uremia. Blood 30:331, 1967.

INDEX

199